T0353589

Practical Case Studies in Hypertension Management

Series editor
Giuliano Tocci
Rome, Italy

The aim of the book series "Practical Case Studies in Hypertension Management" is to provide physicians who treat hypertensive patients having different cardiovascular risk profiles with an easy-to-access tool that will enhance their clinical practice, improve average blood pressure control, and reduce the incidence of major hypertension-related complications. To achieve these ambitious goals, each volume presents and discusses a set of paradigmatic clinical cases relating to different scenarios in hypertension. These cases will serve as a basis for analyzing best practice and highlight problems in implementing the recommendations contained in international guidelines regarding diagnosis and treatment. While the available guidelines have contributed significantly in improving the diagnostic process, cardiovascular risk stratification, and therapeutic management in patients with essential hypertension, they are of relatively limited help to physicians in daily clinical practice when approaching individual patients with hypertension, and this is particularly true when choosing among different drug classes and molecules. By discussing exemplary clinical cases that may better represent clinical practice in a "real world" setting, this series will assist physicians in selecting the best diagnostic and therapeutic options.

More information about this series at http://www.springer.com/series/13624

Massimo Salvetti

Resistant Hypertension

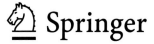 Springer

Prof. Massimo Salvetti
ASST Spedali Civili di Brescia
Clinica Medica-University of Brescia
Brescia, Italy

ISSN 2364-6632   ISSN 2364-6640 (electronic)
Practical Case Studies in Hypertension Management
ISBN 978-3-319-30636-0   ISBN 978-3-319-30637-7 (eBook)
DOI 10.1007/978-3-319-30637-7

Library of Congress Control Number: 2016942889

This Springer imprint is published by Springer Nature
The registered company is Springer International Publishing AG Switzerland

Foreword

Resistant hypertension is a complex clinical condition in which blood pressure levels remained above the recommended targets, despite optimal pharmacological and non-pharmacological treatment. Nowadays, several diagnostic criteria and different therapeutic strategies have been proposed and tested in various clinical settings and study population.

All of these definitions substantially embraced the following aspects: (1) proper assessment of blood pressure levels according to recommendations from international guidelines for measuring blood pressure, (2) optimization of lifestyle changes, (3) exclusion of secondary causes of hypertension, and (4) use of combination therapies at adequate dosages and compounds. Comprehensive and accurate diagnostic evaluation of the potential causes of resistant hypertension represents a crucial aspect for the clinical management of these patients, since several studies have demonstrated that proper lifestyle changes and drug treatment optimization may improve blood pressure control rates and promote the achievement of the recommended blood pressure targets in the majority of patients with apparently resistant hypertension. On the other hand, patients with true resistant hypertension remained at higher risk of major cardiovascular and cerebrovascular complications compared to patients with essential hypertension. As a consequence, these patients with difficult-to-treat hypertension may heavily contribute to the global burden of hypertension-related complications.

In this volume of *Practical Case Studies in Hypertension Management*, the clinical management of paradigmatic cases of patients with resistant hypertension is discussed, focusing on the different diagnostic criteria currently available for properly identifying these high-risk patients, as well as on the different therapeutic options currently recommended for improving blood pressure control and reducing the risk of hypertension-related morbidity and mortality.

Department of Clinical   Giuliano Tocci
and Molecular Medicine
University of Rome Sapienza
St. Andrea Hospital
Rome, Italy

Contents

Clinical Case 1
Adult Patient with True Resistant Hypertension

1.1 Clinical Case Presentation

M. B., a 54-year-old Caucasian female, housemaid, was seen at an office visit for uncontrolled hypertension.

When she was 49, age at which she became menopausal, she was diagnosed as having grade 2 arterial hypertension.

She had been initially treated with a beta blocker, bisoprolol 5 mg OD, and after a few months, an ACE inhibitor had been added (ramipril 5 mg OD) by the general practitioner.

In the following months, the patient was asymptomatic but, according to the patient's description, blood pressure control was not satisfactory.

After 1 year antihypertensive treatment was changed due to poor blood pressure control, and the dose of the ACE inhibitor and of the beta blocker was increased by the general practitioner: ramipril 10 mg once daily and bisoprolol 10 mg were prescribed.

In the following months, blood pressure control was defined as "satisfactory" by the patient.

At the beginning of this year, the patient was seen by the general practitioner for recurrent mild headaches. At the doctor's office, blood pressure was >150/100 mmHg, and hydrochlorothiazide was added, at the dosage of 25 mg once daily.

© Springer International Publishing Switzerland 2016   1
M. Salvetti, *Resistant Hypertension*, Practical
Case Studies in Hypertension Management,
DOI 10.1007/978-3-319-30637-7_1

Family History

Her mother, 78 years old, is hypercholesterolemic. Her father died at the age of 80 for hemorrhagic stroke. She suffered hypertension since the age of 50. She has one brother (50 years old), who is on treatment with statins for hypercholesterolemia, and one sister (51 years old), who is healthy.

She lives with her husband, who is in good health, and they have one daughter.

Clinical History

She has never smoked cigarettes. She does not drink alcohol and has sedentary habits.

She is hypercholesterolemic and is taking simvastatin (20 mg once daily).

She has no other known cardiovascular risk factor, associated clinical conditions or non-cardiovascular diseases.

Physical Examination

- Weight: 86 kg
- Height: 166 cm
- Body mass index (BMI): 31.2 kg/m^2
- Waist circumference: 96 cm
- Respiration: 12/min
- Heart: grade 1 systolic murmur at the apex
- Resting pulse: regular rhythm with normal heart rate (66 beats/min)
- Carotid arteries: no murmurs
- Femoral and foot arteries: palpable
- Clear lungs
- No lower extremity oedema
- The remainder of the examination was normal

Haematological Profile

- Haemoglobin: 14.0 g/dL
- Haematocrit: 44 %
- Fasting plasma glucose: 96 mg/dL
- Fasting lipids: total cholesterol 172 mg/dL; HDL 44 mg/dL; triglycerides 146 mg/dL (LDL, Friedewald formula: 99 mg/dL),
- Electrolytes: sodium, 144 mEq/L; potassium, 3.9 mEq/L
- Serum Uric Acid: 4.9 mg/dL
- Renal function: creatinine, 0.9 mg/dL; estimated glomerular filtration rate (eGFR) (EPI formula: 73 mL/min/1.73 m^2)
- Urine analysis (dipstick): normal
- Urinary albumin excretion: albumin/creatinine ratio 18 mg/g
- Normal liver function tests
- Normal serum TSH

Blood Pressure Profile

Mrs. M.B. was taking measurements of blood pressure values at home on a daily basis, mainly in the afternoon (single measurement).

- Home BP was, on average, 150–155/100 mmHg.
- Office sitting BP: 160/106 mmHg (right arm); 158/104 mmHg (left arm).
- Standing BP: 152/106 mmHg at 1 min.
- 24-h BP: 150/99 mmHg; HR, 63 bpm.
- Daytime BP: 154/101 mmHg; HR, 65 bpm.
- Night-time BP: 143/95 mmHg; HR, 58 bpm.
- The 24-h blood pressure profile may be defined as a "non-dipping pattern" (day/night SBP drop was 7 %). Blood pressure variability was not increased.

The 24-h ambulatory blood pressure profile is illustrated in Fig. 1.1.

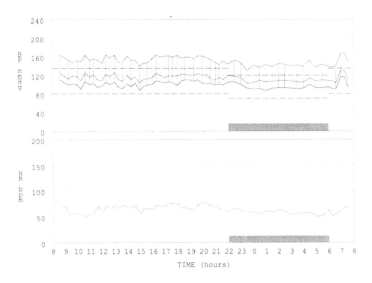

FIGURE 1.1 24-Hour ambulatory blood pressure monitoring

12-Lead Electrocardiogram

The electrocardiogram showed sinus rhythm, without evidence of left ventricular hypertrophy (Cornell voltage <3.5 mV, Cornell product <244 mV*ms, r aVL <1.1 mV).

The repolarization was normal and, in particular, there were no signs of "strain" (Fig. 1.2).

During the visit her husband was asked about the quality of sleep of the partner (snoring, witnessed apneas, restless sleep), and, at the end of the interview, sleep apnoea was judged unlikely in this patient.

Current Treatment

Ramipril 10 mg once daily (h 8:00); bisoprolol 10 mg once daily (h 08.00); hydrochlorothiazide 25 mg (h 8:00).

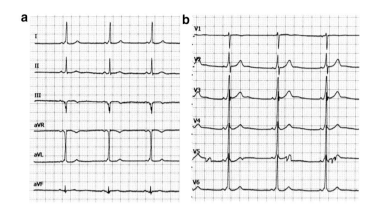

FIGURE 1.2 (**a**, **b**) Electrocardiogram

Diagnosis

– **Resistant hypertension**: arterial hypertension (grade 2) with unsatisfactory BP control despite combination therapy with three drugs
– Central obesity (grade 1, BMI 31)
– Hypercholesterolemia
– Sedentary habits
– No evidence of hypertension-related organ damage or associated clinical conditions.

Which is the global cardiovascular risk profile in this patient?

Possible answers are:

1. Low
2. Medium
3. Moderate to high
4. High

According to ESH ESC 2013 Guidelines CV, added risk is moderate to high [1].

Which is the best therapeutic option in this patient?
Possible answers are:

1. Add another drug.
2. Renal denervation.
3. Reinforce lifestyle changes.
4. Reinforce lifestyle changes and exclude secondary hypertension.

Treatment Evaluation

✓ Ongoing treatment with ACE inhibitor, beta blocker and diuretic was temporarily stopped due to possible interference with aldosterone and renin levels.
✓ Verapamil slow release 120 twice daily was started.
✓ Doxazosin 4 mg OD, in the evening, was started.

Prescriptions

✓ Sampling for plasma renin activity and aldosterone was scheduled, after at least 4 weeks of wash out from the ongoing treatment.
✓ Dosage of 24 h urinary cortisol.
✓ An echocardiogram was also prescribed, with the main aim of evaluating left ventricular structure and function and left atrial size.
✓ The patient was instructed to increase physical activity (mild intensity, at least 4 days weekly) and to reduce caloric and salt intake.

The patient was also advised to contact the doctor in case of severe blood pressure elevation (grade 3 hypertension).

1.2   Follow-Up (Visit 1) at 5 Weeks

At follow-up visit the patient was fine.

She had measured her blood pressure on a daily basis, and mean home BP values were (on average) 150/94 mmHg.

She had started mild physical activity three times per week with initial positive effects (weight loss – 2 kg).

No adverse reactions or drug-related side effects were reported.

Physical Examination

- Weight: 84 kg
- BMI: 30.48 kg/m^2
- Resting pulse: regular rhythm with normal heart rate (66 beats/min)
- Other clinical parameters substantially unchanged

Blood Pressure Profile

- Home BP (average): 150/94 mmHg (mean of measurements in the morning and in the evening)
- Office sitting BP: 158/98 mmHg (left arm)
- Standing BP: 152/98 mmHg (after 1 min)

Current Treatment

✓ Verapamil slow release 120 twice daily
✓ Doxazosin 4 mg OD, in the evening

Aldosterone, Renin and Cortisol Levels

- Aldosterone: 140 pg/mL
- Renin: 6 μUI/mL
- Aldosterone/renin ratio: 2.3
- Urinary cortisol: normal

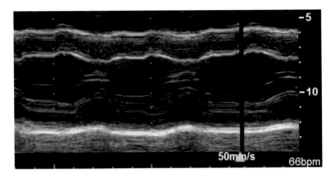

FIGURE 1.3 Echocardiogram showing left ventricular hypertrophy

Echocardiogram

The echocardiogram showed normal left ventricular internal dimensions with an increase in left ventricular mass and an increase in relative wall thickness: **left ventricular hypertrophy, concentric type** (LV mass index, 54 g/m$^{2.7}$; relative wall thickness, 0.53). Preserved endocardial systolic function, reduced midwall fractional shortening. The evaluation of Doppler indices of diastolic function with both conventional and tissue Doppler showed impaired LV relaxation (isovolumic relaxation time 110 ms), without signs of increased LV filling pressure (E/Em 8). Left atrial size and the dimensions of the proximal aorta were normal. Mild mitral regurgitation was observed (+) (Fig. 1.3).

Ultrasound Scan of the Carotid Arteries, with Echo Colour Doppler

Small plaques on the carotid bifurcations. No stenosis (Fig. 1.4)

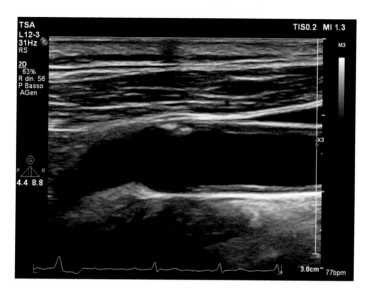

FIGURE 1.4 Echo colour Doppler of the carotid arteries

Diagnosis

Primary aldosteronism?

1. Yes
2. No

The aldosterone/renin was 2.3, which is below the suggested thresholds (<3.7) [5], and furthermore, absolute aldosterone levels were not elevated (<150 pg/mL); therefore, primary aldosteronism was excluded. Urinary cortisol was also within the normal range. Furthermore, there was no evidence of renal artery stenosis or renal disease and there were no sleep disturbances.

Therefore, a final diagnosis was made:

– Essential hypertension, resistant to treatment
– Grade 2, high-added cardiovascular risk

– Cardiac preclinical organ damage (concentric LV hypertrophy), impaired LV diastolic relaxation preclinical vascular damage.
– Abdominal obesity

Treatment Evaluation

✓ Treatment with calcium channel blocker was maintained, switching to a potent dihydropyridine at full dosage.
✓ A long-acting angiotensin receptor blocker was added, at full dosage.
✓ A potent thiazide-like diuretic was added.

Prescribed Treatment

– Olmesartan 40+ amlodipine 10 mg fixed combination once daily at 08.00 am
– Chlortalidone 25 mg once daily at 08.00 am

Prescriptions

✓ Periodical BP evaluation at home according to recommendations from current guidelines
✓ Control of renal function (high-dose diuretic and ARB)
✓ Regular physical activity and low caloric intake

1.3   Follow-Up (Visit 2) at 3 Months

At follow-up visit the patient is fine.

She is following a healthier diet and she performs regular physical activity, three or four times per week. Her weight is improved (– 6 kg from the first visit).

She expresses her preference for fixed (single pill) combination of antihypertensive drugs.

• Electrolytes: sodium, 144 mEq/L; potassium, 3.5 mEq/L
• Serum uric acid: 5.0 mg/dL
• Renal function: creatinine, 0.9 mg/dL; estimated glomerular filtration rate (eGFR) (EPI formula, 70 mL/min/1.73 m^2)

Physical Examination

- Weight: 80 kg
- BMI: 29 kg/m^2
- Waist circumference: 89 cm
- Resting pulse: regular rhythm with 72 beats/min
- Other parameters substantially unchanged

Blood Pressure Profile

- Home BP (average): 140/90 mmHg (early morning)
- Sitting BP: 148/88 mmHg (mean of three measurements, in sitting position)
- Standing BP: 144/92 mmHg

Current Treatment

- Olmesartan 40+ amlodipine 10 mg fixed combination once daily at 08.00 am; chlortalidone 25 mg once daily at 08.00 am

Treatment Evaluation

✓ Spironolactone 25 mg once daily was added.
✓ The combination of ARB, diuretic and calcium antagonist was maintained.

Prescriptions

✓ Periodical BP evaluation at home according to recommendations from current guidelines
✓ Periodical control of creatinine, sodium and potassium with first blood sampling at 3 weeks (use of potassium sparing diuretic)

✓ Regular follow-up visits at the office of the general practitioner (if BP not well controlled, further evaluation at the hypertension clinic, after at least 6 weeks of treatment and lifestyle changes)

1.4   Follow-Up (Visit 2) at 1 Year

After 1 year the patient came to the hypertension clinic for a follow-up visit.

She is frequently seen by her family doctor.

She is in good clinical conditions.

She is maintaining a healthy lifestyle (physical activity four times weekly); her diet is rich in fruit and vegetables, poor in salt.

She understands the importance of antihypertensive treatment for cardiovascular risk reduction.

Physical Examination

- Weight: 75 kg
- Body mass index (BMI): 27 kg/m^2
- Waist circumference: 85 cm
- Resting pulse: regular rhythm with 66 beats/min
- Other parameters substantially unchanged

Blood Pressure Profile

- Home BP (average): 130/80 mmHg
- Sitting BP: 136/82 mmHg
- Standing BP: 132/86 mmHg

12-Lead Electrocardiogram

Sinus rhythm with normal heart rate, normal atrioventricular and intraventricular conduction and no ST-segment abnormalities or signs of LVH without signs of LVH.

Current Treatment

- Olmesartan 40+ amlodipine 10 mg fixed combination once daily at 08.00 am
- Chlortalidone 25 mg once daily at 08.00 am
- Spironolactone 25 mg once daily at 16.00 pm

Treatment Evaluation

✓ No changes for current pharmacological therapy

Prescriptions

✓ Periodical BP evaluation at home according to recommendations from current guidelines.
✓ Regular physical activity and low caloric intake.
✓ Repeat 24-h ambulatory blood pressure monitoring to confirm BP control.
✓ Control of an echocardiogram in the next 6–12 months to evaluate the effect of treatment on LV mass and function (regression of LVH confirms that the prescribed regimen is effective and identifies patients at lower cardiovascular risk, as compared to non-regressors, independently of other CV risk factors).

1.5   Discussion

Resistant hypertension is defined by the 2013 ESH ESC Hypertension Guidelines as a systolic or a diastolic blood pressure that remains above goal (i.e. >140/90 mm Hg for most patients), despite adherence to lifestyle measures and to pharmacological treatment with full doses of at least three antihypertensive medications, including one diuretic [1].

Older age, black race, female sex, obesity, sedentary habits, excess intake of salt and/or alcohol, diabetes, metabolic syndrome, kidney disease and long-standing, poorly controlled hypertension are associated with resistance [2].

Resistant hypertension is recognized as a clinical phenotype carrying a high cardiovascular risk [3]. The increase in cardiovascular risk is likely mediated by uncontrolled blood pressure and frequent comorbidities such as obesity, sleep apnoea, diabetes and target organ damage (renal disease, LVH and cardiovascular disease). The relationship between resistant hypertension and cardiovascular disease/target organ damage may be bidirectional: resistant hypertension may directly cause the development and worsening of target organ damage, through the persistent elevation of blood pressure. The other way around, the presence of cardiovascular target organ damage may contribute to worsen the resistance to treatment, rendering hypertension more difficult to control [4].

This clinical case describes a typical case of true resistant hypertension. In fact BP control was not obtained despite lifestyle changes and a well-designed therapeutic strategy based on the rationale combination of drugs with synergistic effect at full doses. The finding of concentric left ventricular hypertrophy and impaired relaxation at echocardiography further supports the possibility of long-standing, poor blood pressure control and indicates a high cardiovascular risk in this patient [4].

Treatment of true resistant hypertension is challenging. After a correct diagnostic workup [1, 2, 4, 5], the treatment strategy should be tailored to the patient, but, in general, it should include a full-dose diuretic, an ACE inhibitor or an angiotensin receptor blocker and a calcium antagonist, in the absence of compelling indications for other drugs. Mrs. M.B. was treated with chlortalidone, a thiazide-like diuretic. Some, but not all, authors believe that a thiazide-like diuretic, and not hydrochlorotiazide, should be prescribed to patients with resistant hypertension. In fact, it has been postulated that hydrochlorothiazide might be less effective in reducing blood pressure (and, possibly also cardiovascular events) as compared to thiazide-like diuretics such as chlortalidone or indapamide. A recent meta-analysis, based on head-to-head comparisons of the two types of diuretics, supports a greater antihypertensive effect of thiazide-like diuretics, but it must be admitted that no definitive conclusion may be drawn, since no large, randomized study has been designed with this purpose [6].

When true resistant hypertension is diagnosed, the choice of the fourth drug should be based on the clinical characteristics of the patient, since data based on randomized trials are scanty [1]. Spironolactone is gaining success as a fourth drug in patients with resistant hypertension, due to the efficacy in reducing blood pressure values, as demonstrated in a post hoc analysis in the ASCOT study population [7]. In patients without primary aldosteronism, the blood pressure response to antialdosterone drugs may be accounted for by the elevated plasma aldosterone levels frequently accompanying resistant hypertension, because aldosterone secretion escapes the early reduction associated with RAS blockade.

Very recently the results of the "Optimal Treatment of Drug Resistant Hypertension-PATHWAY 2" trial have been presented at the Congress of the European Society of Cardiology and published in Lancet [8]. Treatment with spironolactone resulted unequivocally superior to the other therapeutic strategies tested, which were based on the beta-blocker bisoprolol and the α-blocker doxazosin.

Take-Home Messages

- Resistant hypertension is defined by the 2013 ESH ESC Hypertension Guidelines as a systolic or a diastolic blood pressure that remains above goal, despite adherence to lifestyle measures and to pharmacological treatment with full doses of at least three antihypertensive medications, possibly including one diuretic.
- True resistant hypertension is a condition characterized by high cardiovascular risk.
- Treatment strategies should be based on well-designed combinations of antihypertensive drugs with synergistic effect at full doses.

(continued)

Take-Home Messages (continued)

- The combination of drugs, in most cases, should include a full-dose diuretic, an ACE inhibitor or an angiotensin receptor blocker and a calcium antagonist, in the absence of compelling indications for different drugs.
- As fourth drug, good response has been reported to the use of mineralocorticoid receptor antagonists, i.e. spironolactone, even at low doses (25–50 mg/day) and with the alpha-1-blocker doxazosin.
- Very recent data give further support to the use of antialdosterone drugs as fourth drug in these patients. However, it must be kept in mind that the use of antialdosterone drugs requires frequent monitoring of creatinine and electrolytes.

References

1. Mancia G, Fagard R, Narkiewicz K, Redon J, Zanchetti A, Bohm M, et al. 2013 ESH/ESC Guidelines for the management of arterial hypertension: the Task Force for the management of arterial hypertension of the European Society of Hypertension (ESH) and of the European Society of Cardiology (ESC). J Hypertens. 2013;31(7):1281–357.
2. Calhoun DA, Jones D, Textor S, Goff DC, Murphy TP, Toto RD, et al. Resistant hypertension: diagnosis, evaluation, and treatment. A scientific statement from the American Heart Association Professional Education Committee of the Council for High Blood Pressure Research. Circulation. 2008;117:e510–26.
3. Daugherty SL, Powers JD, Magid DJ, Tavel HM, Masoudi FA, Margolis KL, O'Connor PJ, Selby JV, Ho PM. Incidence and prognosis of resistant hypertension in hypertensive patients. Circulation. 2012;125:1635–42.

4. Muiesan ML, Salvetti M, Rizzoni D, Paini A, Agabiti-Rosei C, Aggiusti C, Agabiti Rosei E. Resistant hypertension and target organ damage. Hypertens Res. 2013;36(6):485–91.
5. Funder JW, Carey RM, Fardella C, Gomez-Sanchez CE, Mantero F, Stowasser M, Young Jr WF, Montori VM, Endocrine Society. Case detection, diagnosis, and treatment of patients with primary aldosteronism: an endocrine society clinical practice guideline. J Clin Endocrinol Metab. 2008;93(9):3266–81.
6. Roush GC, Ernst ME, Kostis JB, Tandon S, Sica DA. Head-to-head comparisons of hydrochlorothiazide with indapamide and chlorthalidone: antihypertensive and metabolic effects. Hypertension. 2015;65(5):1041–6.
7. Chapman N, Dobson J, Wilson S, et al. Effect of spironolactone on blood pressure in subjects with resistant hypertension. Hypertension. 2007;49:839–45.
8. Williams B, MacDonald TM, Morant S, Webb DJ, Sever P, McInnes G, Ford I, Cruickshank JK, Caulfield MJ, Salsbury J, Mackenzie I, Padmanabhan S, Brown MJ, British Hypertension Society's PATHWAY Studies Group. Spironolactone versus placebo, bisoprolol, and doxazosin to determine the optimal treatment for drug-resistant hypertension (PATHWAY-2): a randomised, double-blind, crossover trial. Lancet. 2015;386: 2059–68.

Clinical Case 2

Adult Patient with Pseudo-Resistant Hypertension: High Blood Pressure Induced by Exogenous Substances

2.1 Clinical Case Presentation

A. A., female, 28 years, Caucasian, laboratory technician, came to the echolab of the Hypertension Clinic with the prescription for an echocardiogram and an ultrasound scan of the carotid arteries for the assessment of hypertensive preclinical organ damage.

She was taking levothyroxine for primary hypothyroidism due to Hashimoto's thyroiditis.

She had been visited about 2 months before by her endocrinologist for mild headaches and recent onset (5 days) hypertension. At the time of the first visit at the endocrinologist's office, blood pressure (BP) values were 210/120 mmHg (sitting, after 3 min of rest). Amlodipine 10 mg OD had been prescribed to the patient; self-measurement of blood pressure had also been recommended, together with a strict follow-up at the practitioner office.

After 10 days BP values were unchanged, and enalapril 20/hydrochlorothiazide 12.5 mg fixed combination had been added (dose increased to 20/12.5×2).

After other 2 weeks, BP values were unchanged. The specialist had planned a complete workup for secondary hypertension. A renal ultrasound scan with echo Doppler evaluation of the renal arteries was normal. The ACE inhibitor and the

© Springer International Publishing Switzerland 2016
M. Salvetti, *Resistant Hypertension*, Practical
Case Studies in Hypertension Management,
DOI 10.1007/978-3-319-30637-7_2

diuretic had been stopped, due to apparent inefficacy and to the possible interference with aldosterone and renin dosage.

Family History

Her mother, 58 years old, was in good health. Her father was hypercholesterolemic. She was a single child. She lives alone.

Clinical History

She does not drink alcohol and is physically active. She smokes about ten cigarettes per day.

No other known cardiovascular risk factor, associated clinical conditions or non-cardiovascular diseases.

Physical Examination

- Weight: 46 kg
- Height: 158 cm
- Body mass index (BMI): 18.4 kg/m^2
- Respiration: 11/min
- Heart: normal
- Resting pulse: regular rhythm with normal heart rate (72 beats/min)
- Carotid arteries: no murmurs
- Femoral and foot arteries: palpable
- Clear lungs
- No lower extremity oedema
- Remainder of the examination: normal

Haematological Profile

- Haemoglobin: 12.3 g/dL
- Haematocrit: 38 %
- Fasting plasma glucose: 82 mg/dL

- Fasting lipids: total cholesterol 176 mg/dL; HDL 58 mg/dL; triglycerides 115 mg/dL (LDL, Friedewald formula: 95 mg/dL)
- Electrolytes: sodium, 143 mEq/L; potassium, 3.3 mEq/L (normal values of the lab: 3.3–4.7)
- Serum uric acid: 3.9 mg/dL
- Renal function: creatinine, 0.6 mg/dL; estimated glomerular filtration rate (eGFR) (EPI formula: 125 mL/min/1.73 m^2)
- Urine analysis (dipstick): normal
- Urinary albumin excretion: albumin/creatinine ratio 16 mg/g
- Normal liver function tests
- Normal serum TSH

Blood Pressure Profile

When she came to the echolab of the hypertension clinic, Mrs A. A. had started taking measurements of blood pressure values at home every day, in the morning before breakfast and in the evening before dinner; she had been instructed to record the mean value of 2–3 measurements.

- Home BP was, on average, 150/100 mmHg.
- Office sitting BP: 155/110 mmHg (right arm); 152/110 mmHg (left arm).
- Standing BP: 148/112 mmHg at 1 min.

The ambulatory blood pressure monitoring profile showed a stable increase in BP values over 24 h, with values largely above the suggested thresholds both during the day and the night.

- 24-h BP: 155/111 mmHg; HR: 71 bpm
- Daytime BP: 160/116 mmHg; HR: 74 bpm
- Night-time BP: 143/100 mmHg; HR: 67 bpm

Overall, the results of the ABPM showed a severe increase of BP values. The reduction of BP during night-time was borderline (day/night SBP drop was 10.5 %).

The 24-h ambulatory blood pressure tracing is illustrated in Fig. 2.1.

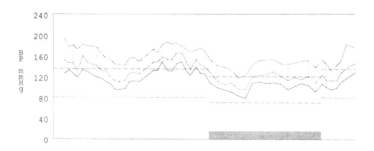

FIGURE 2.1 24-hour blood pressure profile

12-Lead Electrocardiogram

The electrocardiogram was normal (sinus rhythm; Cornell voltage <3.5 mV, Cornell product <244 mV ms, r aVL <1.1 mV).
    The repolarization was normal.

Fundoscopic Examination

An ophthalmological evaluation for the assessment of hypertensive retinal changes was urgently performed. The exam was substantially normal.

Current Treatment

Amlodipine 10 mg once daily (h 8:00).

Diagnosis

The patient was seen at the echolab with the provisional diagnosis of:
– **Severe (grade 3) new onset hypertension** (suspect secondary hypertension, workup in progress).
– Primary hypothyroidism due to Hashimoto's thyroiditis.

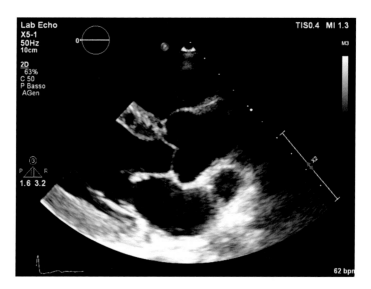

FIGURE 2.2   Echocardiogram: parasternal long axis view

Echocardiogram.

The echocardiogram showed normal left ventricular (LV) internal dimensions (end diastolic diameter 4.7 cm) and **normal left ventricular mass and geometry** (septum thickness 0.94 cm, posterior wall 0.75 cm, LV mass 116 g, LVMI index 83 g/m^2 and 34 g/m$^{2.7}$; relative wall thickness 0.34) (Fig. 2.2). Preserved endocardial, midwall and longitudinal systolic function. Left ventricular ejection fraction was 55 %. The evaluation of Doppler indices of diastolic function with both conventional and tissue Doppler showed a normal pattern (E/A ratio 1.6, E dec t 210 ms, isovolumic relaxation time 88 ms), without signs of increased LV filling pressure (E/Em 7.4) (Fig. 2.3). Left atrial size: linear dimension (parasternal) 3 cm, volume 27 ml/m^2.

– Aorta: tricuspid valve, normal dimensions (Fig. 2.4).
– Mild mitral and tricuspid regurgitation were observed (+). Pulmonary artery systolic pressure 24 mmHg.

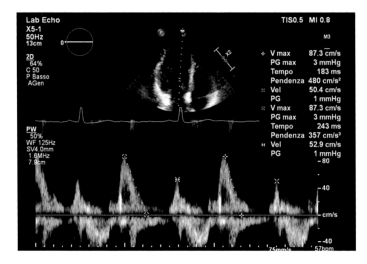

FIGURE 2.3 Echocardiogram: transmitral flow

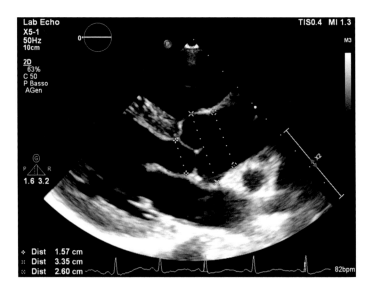

FIGURE 2.4 Echocardiogram: aortic size

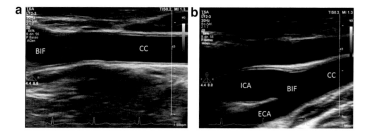

Figure 2.5 (**a**, **b**) Carotid artery ultrasound. *CC*, common carotid; *BIF*, carotid bifurcation; *ICA*, internal carotid artery; *ECA*, external carotid artery

Ultrasound Evaluation of the Carotid Arteries

Normal intima media thickness at the level of the common carotid artery, of the bifurcation and internal carotid arteries, bilaterally. Vertebral arteries: normal flow (Fig. 2.5).

> **Which is the global cardiovascular risk profile in this patient?**
> Possible answers are:
>
> 1. Low
> 2. Medium
> 3. High
> 4. Very high

Cardiovascular risk according to ESH ESC 2013 Guidelines is high; in this case the level of risk is driven by the very high BP levels and not by other risk factors, organ damage or comorbidities.

During the preliminary clinical history at the echolab of the hypertension clinic, the patient showed the first results of the hormonal tests ordered by the endocrinologist (sample after wash out from ACE inhibitor +diuretic):

Plasma aldosterone (orthostatism): <37 pg/ml
Plasma renin (orthostatism): <5 μUI/ml
Urinary cortisol (24 h): 20 mcg
Urinary metanephrines: ongoing

During the preliminary clinical history at the echolab of the hypertension clinic, the medical staff asked about the use of illicit drugs, other substances and in particular of liquorice or nasal spray.

The patient admitted to have started eating liquorice candies on a daily basis about 1 month ago.

Treatment Evaluation

✓ Ongoing treatment with amlodipine was continued.
✓ Doxazosin 1 mg was administered; the patient was pre-scribed to take an additional dose of 2 mg in the evening (with measurement of BP before drug intake) and subsequently 2 mg at 8 pm and 2 mg at 20 pm with frequent BP measurements.
✓ The patient was asked to stop the consumption of liquorice candies (advice about the possible harms and the possible severe elevation of BP associated with intake of large amounts of liquorice was given).

Prescriptions

✓ Measurement of BP values at least three times in a day
✓ The patient was sent back to the endocrinologist office for adjustment of antihypertensive treatment (i.e. reduction/ withdrawal in case of BP reduction, increase if inadequate BP control)

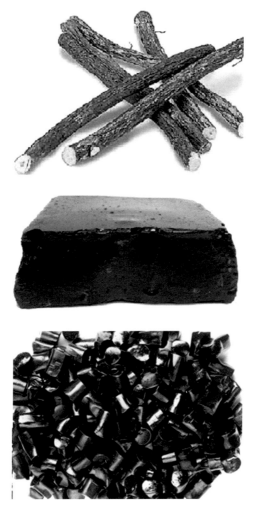

FIGURE 2.6   Various forms of liquorice that can be found in the market

2.2   Follow-Up (Visit 1) at the Endocrinologist's Office (1 Day After the Echocardiogram and After Initiation of Doxazosin)

Headache had disappeared.

She had measured her blood pressure in the previous evening (150/100 mmHg) and the same morning of the visit (140/90 mmHg).

No adverse reactions or drug-related side effects were reported.

Physical Examination

- Unchanged
- Resting pulse: regular rhythm with normal heart rate (76 beats/min)

Current Treatment

✓ Amlodipine 10 mg once daily, in the morning
✓ Doxazosin 2 mg OD taken the evening before the visit

Treatment Evaluation

✓ Treatment with calcium channel blocker was maintained; advice was given to halve the dose of amlodipine if BP < 140/90 mmHg, anticipating a possible reduction of BP with the cessation of liquorice assumption.
✓ Doxazosin 2 mg OD was maintained, until waiting for the results of the metanephrines.

Prescriptions

✓ Measurement of BP values at least three times in a day. Follow up for the next days at the GP office.

2.3 Follow-Up (Visit 2) (4 Days After the Echocardiogram)

The patient had reduced amlodipine to 5 mg OD in the morning and doxazosin to 1 mg OD in the evening.

Physical Examination

- Unchanged
- Resting pulse: regular rhythm with 90 beats/min
- Other parameters substantially unchanged

Blood Pressure Profile

- Home BP (average): 95/60 mmHg
- Sitting BP in the office: 90/60 mmHg (mean of three measurements, in sitting position)
- Standing BP: 86/66 mmHg, HR 100 bpm

Current Treatment

- Amlodipine 5 mg OD
- Doxazosin 1 mg OD

Treatment Evaluation

✓ Treatment was stopped.
✓ Laboratory was contacted: the preliminary results of the dosage of metanephrines were as follows:

Adrenaline: <0.03 mg/24 h.
Noradrenaline: 0.048 mg/24 h.
Dopamine: 0.144 mg/24 h.
Metanephrine: 0.102 mg/24 h.
Normetanephrine: 0.291 mg/24 h.
3-Methoxytyramine: 0.091 mg/24 h.
Therefore, a pheochromocytoma was definitely excluded (as expected).

Diagnosis

A diagnosis was made:

– **Severe (grade 3), transient, treatment-resistant hypertension, secondary to ingestion of large doses of liquorice**
– Primary hypothyroidism due to Hashimoto's thyroiditis

Prescriptions

✓ The patient was instructed to avoid ingestion of liquorice.
✓ Measurement of BP at home in the next weeks was
recommended.
✓ Follow up at the GP office.

2.4   Follow-Up (Visit 3, Final Visit)
at 1 Month

The patient is in good clinical conditions.
   She is maintaining a healthy lifestyle, she does not eat
liquorice candies, but she is still smoking ten cigarettes per
day.

• Weight: 46.5 kg
• Height: 158 cm
• Body mass index (BMI): 18.6 kg/m^2
• Respiration: 10/min
• Heart: normal
• Resting pulse: regular rhythm with normal heart rate
(80 beats/min)
• Carotid arteries: no murmurs
• Femoral and foot arteries: palpable
• Clear lungs
• No lower extremity oedema
• Remainder of the examination: normal

Blood Pressure Profile

- Home BP (average): 90/68 mmHg
- Sitting BP: 94/72 mmHg
- Standing BP: 92/78 mmHg

12-Lead Electrocardiogram

Not performed (not appropriate).

Current Treatment

- No treatment

Treatment Evaluation

✓ No treatment

Prescriptions

✓ Smoking cessation
✓ Regular physical activity
✓ Healthy diet

Diagnosis

A final diagnosis was made:

- **Severe (grade 3), transient, treatment-resistant hyper-tension, secondary to ingestion of large doses of liquorice**
- **Complete resolution of the hypertensive state after withdrawal of liquorice**
- Primary hypothyroidism due to Hashimoto's thyroiditis

2.5   Discussion

Resistant hypertension is not uncommon, with a reported prevalence between 5 and 30 % depending on the population examined (10 % is probably the most appropriate estimate) [1, 2]. However, in most cases, an appropriate approach may reveal reversible factors responsible for poor BP control. In patients referred for resistant hypertension, the diagnostic workup should include the evaluation of possible secondary forms of hypertension. Particular attention should be paid to the possible effect of several classes of pharmacological agents on BP, since they could significantly contribute to treatment resistance in these patients [1, 2].

In this clinical case, a young patient had developed arterial hypertension in an apparently short time window. This raised strong suspects of secondary hypertension. In this case, however, doctors should also consider alternative explanations, such as the possibility that BP elevation could have been induced by drugs or exogenous substances [1]. The attending endocrinologist in the initial workup did not pay sufficient attention to this aspect. Patients often ignore the possible effect of substances or drugs on BP values and should therefore be specifically asked about the intake of drugs, liquorice and nasal sprays [1–6]. Due to the sudden and severe elevation of BP values, the attending endocrinologist ordered also dosage of urinary metanephrines, which are considered the best initial test when pheochromocytoma is suspected, due to a very high sensitivity (>97 %) [7].

In the case presented here, ingestion of large amounts of liquorice (Fig. 2.6) led to severe, treatment-resistant hypertension. In ancient times Egyptians, Babylonians, Greeks, Romans, Brahmans of India and Chinese used liquorice for medical purposes (Hippocrates used liquorice to heal wounds and sore throats) as well as for its pleasant taste. It is derived from the root of *Glycyrrhiza*, a genus of about 18 species in the legume family of Fabaceae (Fig. 2.7). Glycyrrhetinic acid inhibits, both competitively and by reducing gene expression, 11-beta-HSD2, the same enzyme that is deficient in patients with the apparent mineralocorticoid excess syndrome

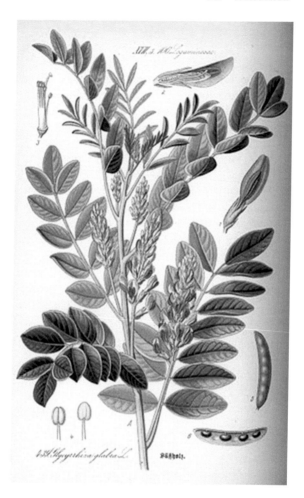

FIGURE 2.7 *Glycyrrhiza glabra*

(AME), a rare genetic form of severe hypertension [4, 5]. Therefore, the clinical picture may resemble that of AME: including hypertension, muscle weakness, hypokalaemia, low plasma renin activity and low plasma aldosterone levels or some combination of the above. Similar signs and symptoms may also be induced by liquorice-like compounds such as carbenoxolone.

The clinical picture may vary significantly, depending on the concentration of glycyrrhetinic acid, but also by individual characteristic of the patients. Some results seem also to indicate a role for a genetic predisposition to BP increase during exposure to liquorice. The degree of BP elevation may vary between mild elevations of BP values to severe hypertension and, sometimes, hypertensive emergencies [6].

In this patient the absence of cardiac, vascular and renal organ damage supports a relatively short duration of BP elevation. The mechanisms underlying the elevation of BP values became apparent after the interview with the patient at the echolab, but were also indirectly confirmed by the finding of levels of renin and aldosterone particularly low.

The subsequent normalization of BP values further confirmed the aetiology of BP elevation.

Take-Home Messages

- In patients referred for resistant hypertension, an accurate initial workup should always be performed.
- Particular attention should be paid to the possible effect of drugs and/or exogenous substances on BP, since they could significantly contribute to treatment resistance in these patients.
- Ingestion of large amounts of liquorice my lead to severe, treatment-resistant hypertension.
- In these cases, the clinical picture may resemble that of AME, including hypertension, muscle weakness, hypokalaemia, low plasma renin activity and aldosterone levels.
- Cessation of the assumption of liquorice results in normalization of BP.

References

1. Calhoun DA, Jones D, Textor S, Goff DC, Murphy TP, Toto RD, et al. Resistant hypertension: diagnosis, evaluation, and treatment. A scientific statement from the American Heart Association Professional Education Committee of the Council for High Blood Pressure Research. Circulation. 2008;117:e510–26.
2. Mancia G, Fagard R, Narkiewicz K, Redon J, Zanchetti A, Bohm M, et al. 2013 ESH/ESC Guidelines for the management of arterial hypertension: the Task Force for the management of arterial hypertension of the European Society of Hypertension (ESH) and of the European Society of Cardiology (ESC). J Hypertens. 2013;31(7):1281–357.
3. Farese Jr RV, Biglieri EG, Shackleton CH, et al. Licorice induced hypermineralocorticoidism. N Engl J Med. 1991;325(17):1223–7.
4. Walker BR, Edwards CR. Licorice-induced hypertension and syndromes of apparent mineralocorticoid excess. Endocrinol Metab Clin North Am. 1994;23(2):359–77.
5. Miettinen HE, Piippo K, Hannila-Handelberg T, Paukku K, Hiltunen TP, Gautschi I, Schild L, Kontula K. Licorice-induced hypertension and common variants of genes regulating renal sodium reabsorption. Ann Med. 2010;42(6):465–74. doi:10.3109/0 7853890.2010.499133.
6. Schröder T, Hubold C, Muck P, Lehnert H, Haas CS. A hypertensive emergency with acute visual impairment due to excessive liquorice consumption. Neth J Med. 2015;73(2):82–5.
7. Lenders J, Duh Q, Eisenhofer G, Gimenez-Roqueplo A, Grebe S, Murad M, Naruse M, Pacak K, Young W. Pheochromocytoma and paraganglioma: an endocrine society clinical practice guideline. J Clin Endocrinol Metab. 2014;99:1915–42.

Clinical Case 3
Adult Patient with Pseudo-Resistant Hypertension: Low Adherence

3.1 Clinical Case Presentation

P. V., a 57-year-old Caucasian male, business consultant, came to the hypertension clinic for a visit.

One month before, when he was on holiday, he had been admitted to the ED of a local hospital for chest pain. A coronary angiography had been performed, due to the presence of chest pain, ECG changes and borderline troponin I values. The coronary arteries were almost normal. Renal arteries were also evaluated at the same time by angiography (normal findings). Grade 3 blood pressure (BP) values were recorded (220/110 mmHg).

Family History

His father died at the age of 55 for gastric cancer and was hypertensive. His mother, 79 years old, is affected by reflux oesophagitis. He has one sister (49 years old), who is on treatment with statins for hypercholesterolemia. He lives with his wife, who is in good health, and they have one healthy daughter.

© Springer International Publishing Switzerland 2016   37
M. Salvetti, *Resistant Hypertension*, Practical
Case Studies in Hypertension Management,
DOI 10.1007/978-3-319-30637-7_3

Clinical History

He smokes cigarettes (at least 20 cigarettes per day since when he was 18 years old). He drinks alcohol (he declares to drink about 1 l of wine every day and, "occasionally", some hard drinks).

He is not particularly active but not sedentary; his diet is rich in meat and salt, poor in vegetables.

He complains mild erectile dysfunction and occasionally uses sildenafil.

Arterial hypertension has been detected for the first time about 1 year before the visit. At that time, he had experienced mild palpitations and had measured blood pressure with the automated device of a friend, obtaining a reading of 220/120 mmHg. He had been admitted to the ED of a small hospital where grade 3 hypertension had been confirmed (200/110 mmHg), with moderately elevated creatinine values (1.5 mg/dL, normal potassium). Despite this the patient had refused to initiate antihypertensive treatment for months. Three months before the visit, he had started treatment with ramipril 5 mg+ hydrochlorotiazide 25 mg. One month before the visit, he had started also atenolol (50 mg OD initially, subsequently increased to 50 mg in the morning + 50 mg in the evening).

The patient was substantially asymptomatic, but, during the last weeks, the sudden death of a friend had focused his attention on BP values, after a long period in which he had almost ignored the problem.

In a recent visit at the office of the medical practitioner, the recorded values were around 160/100 mmHg.

Previous diseases are tibial plateau fracture and laparoscopic cholecystectomy; there are no other known cardiovascular risk factors, associated clinical conditions or non-cardiovascular diseases.

Physical Examination

- Weight: 72 kg
- Height: 178 cm
- Body mass index (BMI): 23 kg/m^2

- Waist circumference: 86 cm
- Respiration: 12/min
- Heart sounds: S1–S2 regular, grade 2 systolic murmur at the apex
- Resting pulse: regular rhythm (70 beats/min)
- Carotid arteries: no murmurs
- Femoral and foot arteries: palpable
- Clear lungs
- No lower extremity oedema
- The remainder of the examination was normal

Haematological Profile

- Haemoglobin: 14.1 g/dL
- Mean corpuscular volume: 92
- WBC $9.1 \times 10^3/\mu L$
- PLT $244 \times 10^3/\mu L$
- Fasting plasma glucose: 99 mg/dL
- Fasting lipids: total cholesterol 202 mg/dL, HDL 42 mg/dL, LDL 125 mg/dL, triglycerides 168 mg/dL
- Electrolytes: sodium, 142 mEq/L; potassium, 3.7 mEq/L
- Serum uric acid: 4.0 mg/dL
- Renal function: creatinine 1.4 mg/dL, eGFR CKD-EPI 55 mL/min/1.73 m^2
- Urine analysis (dipstick): normal
- Albuminuria: albumin/creatinine ratio, not available
- Liver function tests (AST 12 U/L, ALT 18 U/L)
- TSH: not tested

Blood Pressure Profile

Mr P. V. does not measure regularly blood pressure at home; only occasionally he takes a single measurement, when his wife reminds him that he should do it.

The few values reported are well above the suggested cut-off of 135/85 mmHg.

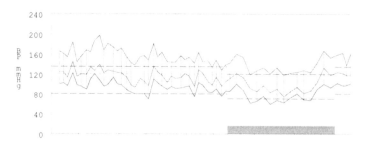

FIGURE 3.1 24-hour blood pressure profile

- Office sitting BP: 160/96 mmHg; no difference between arms. Heart rate 80 r
- Standing BP: 156/100 mmHg at 1 min

The ambulatory blood pressure monitoring profile shows increased 24 h BP values, with values above the suggested thresholds both during the day and the night.

- 24-h BP: 149/89 mmHg; HR: 80 bpm
- Daytime BP: 157/95 mmHg; HR: 81 bpm
- Night-time BP: 137/78 mmHg; HR: 78 bpm

Therefore, 24 h BP values are definitely above the thresholds proposed by the ESH Guidelines (24 h < 135/85 mmHg). Furthermore, both daytime and night-time BP values are elevated.

The analysis of 24-h blood pressure profile shows an increased BP variability, as indicated by the standard deviation of BP values (standard deviation of 24 h SBP, 18.10; standard deviation of night-time SBP, 15.79).

Day-to-night BP reduction was 13 %.

The 24-h ambulatory blood pressure profile is illustrated in Fig. 3.1.

12-Lead Electrocardiogram

The electrocardiogram showed sinus rhythm and left ventricular hypertrophy with a strain pattern (Fig. 3.2).

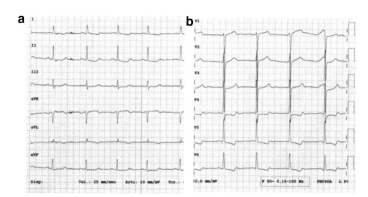

FIGURE 3.2 Electrocardiogram

Echocardiogram

The echocardiogram showed concentric left ventricular hypertrophy (LVMI 59 g/m$^{2.7}$, RWT 0.55), with preserved systolic function. Left atrial volume was the upper limits of normality (33 mL/BSA). It also showed delayed relaxation and possible increase in LV filling pressures (IVRT 125 ms, TDI: E/E^1 13.0).

Vascular Ultrasound

A carotid ultrasound scan (with pulsed and colour Doppler) was performed. The exam showed small, marginal plaques at the level of the left carotid bifurcation and of the right internal carotid artery (Fig. 3.3).

Arterial Stiffness

Carotid to femoral pulse wave velocity (PWV) was increased (13.6 m/s) (Fig. 3.4).

As already mentioned, the renal arteries had been evaluated about 1 month ago during coronary angiography.

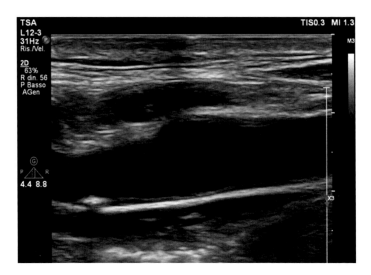

FIGURE 3.3 Carotid ultrasound

An abdominal ultrasound performed about 1 year before was substantially normal.

The wife of the patient was present at the time of the visit and sleep apnoea was ruled out.

Current Treatment

Ramipril 5 mg once daily (h 8:00); hydrochlorothiazide 25 mg (h 8:00); atenolol 50 mg × 2 (h 08.00 and 20.00).

Which is the global cardiovascular risk profile in this patient?

Possible answers are:
1. Low
2. Medium
3. High
4. Very high

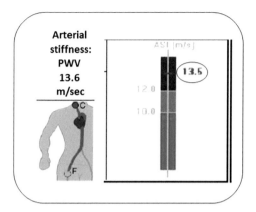

<small>FIGURE 3.4</small> Arterial stiffness: carotid-femoral PWV

Global Cardiovascular Risk Stratification

According to 2013 ESH/ESC global cardiovascular risk stratification [1], this patient has a high cardiovascular risk profile.

Workup

True resistant hypertension was considered possible, but not definitely confirmed. Verapamil slow release 120 twice daily was started; a letter was sent to the medical practitioner, indicating the possibility of adding an alpha blocker during the workup for secondary hypertension in case of significant increase of BP values. A workup for secondary forms of hypertension was programmed.

A long interview with the patient and his wife was carried out, and the risks associated to increased blood pressure values were extensively illustrated. Particular attention was paid to the importance of adherence to antihypertensive treatment.

Furthermore, the importance of lifestyle changes, and in particular of smoking cessation and of the reduction of alcohol consumption, was particularly stressed.

Treatment Evaluation

✓ Ongoing treatment was stopped due to possible interference with hormonal testing.
✓ Verapamil slow release 120 twice daily was started.

Prescriptions

Dosage of aldosterone and plasma renin activity (after at least 3 weeks of washout) and of 24-h urinary cortisol and metanephrines was programmed. Testing for microalbuminuria was also scheduled.

✓ Lifestyle changes were recommended.
✓ Adherence to treatment was also recommended.

3.2   Follow-Up (Visit 1) at 4 Weeks

At follow-up visit, the patient was asymptomatic.

He had started regular measurements of BP values. Mean values at home were, on average, 140–145/90 mmHg.

He had reduced the daily number of cigarettes and had improved his lifestyle by reducing alcohol intake and increasing physical activity (walking, three times per week). Body weight was unchanged.

The patient reported to pay more attention to adherence to antihypertensive treatment and to appreciate the reduction in the number of pills ("I like taking less pills").

No drug-related side effects were reported.

Physical Examination

• Weight: 71.5 kg
• Height: 178 cm

- BMI: 22.7 kg/m^2
- Resting pulse: regular rhythm with normal heart rate (60 beats/min)
- Other clinical parameters substantially unchanged

Blood Pressure Profile

- Home BP (average): 140–145/90 mmHg
- Office sitting BP: 148/96 mmHg
- Standing BP: 144/100 mmHg at 1 min

Current Treatment

✓ Verapamil slow release 120 twice daily

Aldosterone, Renin and Cortisol Levels

- Aldosterone: 100 pg/mL
- Renin: 7 µU/mL
- Aldosterone/renin ratio: 1.4
- Urinary cortisol: normal
- Albumin/creatinine ratio: 42 mg/g

Diagnosis

Which is the correct diagnosis?
Possible answers are:

1. Primary aldosteronism.
2. Essential hypertension.
3. Cushing syndrome.
4. There is suspicion of primary aldosteronism and a confirmatory test is required.

Diagnosis

Essential hypertension with poor adherence to lifestyle measures and with poor compliance to antihypertensive treatment.

There is no evidence of primary aldosteronism, Cushing disease, renovascular hypertension and sleep apnoea syndrome.

It is possible that in this patient reinforcing lifestyle measures and increasing adherence to antihypertensive treatment could lead to a significant reduction of BP values.

Treatment Evaluation

✓ Treatment with a fixed combination of an ACE inhibitor and a calcium antagonist was initiated.

Prescribed Treatment

Perindopril 10 mg/amlodipine 10 mg fixed combination, in the morning.

Prescriptions

✓ Periodical BP evaluation at home according to recommendations from current guidelines.
✓ Control of renal function (high-dose ACE-i).
✓ Regular physical activity and low caloric intake. Smoking cessation.
✓ Adherence to treatment was recommended (further discussion on the importance of adherence to the therapeutic plan in order to maximize cardiovascular protection).

3.3   Follow-Up (Visit 2) at 3 Months

At follow-up visit at 3 months, the patient was in good conditions and asymptomatic.

He was following our recommendations, having increased physical activity, reduced alcohol intake to one drink per day and performing regular physical activity (4–5 days per week). His weight was slightly reduced (–2 kg from the first visit). He smokes 2–4 cigarettes per day.

He is taking regularly his medicines and appreciates the reduced burden of pills.

- Electrolytes: sodium, 143 mEq/L; potassium, 4.4 mEq/L
- Renal function: creatinine 1.35 mg/dL, eGFR CKD-EPI 58 mL/min/1.73 m^2

Physical Examination

- Weight: 70 kg
- BMI: 22.1 kg/m^2
- Resting pulse: regular rhythm with 72 beats/min
- Other parameters substantially unchanged
- No ankle oedema

Blood Pressure Profile

- Home BP (average values during the last week, daily measurements in the morning and evening): 134/80 mmHg (early morning)
- Sitting BP in the office: 138/86 mmHg (mean of three measurements, in sitting position)
- Heart rate 72 bpm
- Standing BP: 138/92 mmHg

Current Treatment

- Perindopril 10/amlodipine 10 fixed-single pill combination at 8 am

Treatment Evaluation

✓ The combination of ACE inhibitor and dihydropiridinic calcium antagonist was maintained.

Prescriptions

✓ The patient was advised to maintain lifestyle measures and to quit smoking.
✓ Home BP measurement was recommended, together with periodic BP measurement at the office of the general practitioner.
✓ Testing for creatinine, potassium, glucose, lipids, urinanalysis and albumin/creatinine ratio before the next visit

3.4   Follow-Up (Visit 2) at 1 Year

At 12 months from the first visit at the hypertension clinic, the patient was in good clinical conditions.

He was continuing physical activity (physical activity 4 times weekly, about 1 h of brisk walking or running), and his diet is rich in fruit and vegetables, poor in salt.

He is still smoking 2–3 cigarettes per day.

He is taking his pills regularly.

Physical Examination

- Weight: 70 kg
- Body mass index (BMI): 22.1 kg/m^2

- Resting pulse: regular rhythm with 72 beats/min
- Remainder of the examination: unremarkable

Haematological Profile

- Fasting plasma glucose: 94 mg/dL
- Fasting lipids: total cholesterol 184 mg/dL, HDL 53 mg/dL, triglycerides 114 mg/dL, LDL (Friedewald formula) 109 mg/dL
- Electrolytes: potassium, 4.6 mEq/L
- Renal function: creatinine, 1.3 mg/dL; estimated glomerular filtration rate (eGFR) (CKD-EPI 61 mL/min/1.73 m^2
- Urine analysis (dipstick): normal
- Albuminuria: albumin/creatinine ratio 20 mg/g

Blood Pressure Profile

- Home BP (average values during the last week): 134/82 mmHg.
- Sitting BP: 138/84 mmHg.
- Standing BP: 138/88 mmHg.
- The patient reported that, during the last week, BP values were measured by the family doctor and were slightly elevated: 145/90 mmHg.

   The electrocardiogram was substantially unchanged.

Current Treatment

- Perindopril 10/amlodipine 10 fixed-single pill combination at 8 a.m.

Treatment Evaluation

✓ Current treatment was left unchanged and an ambulatory blood pressure monitoring was performed.

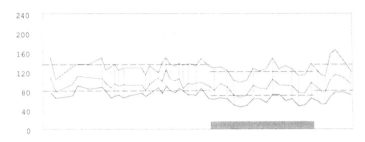

FIGURE 3.5 24-hour blood pressure profile at last visit

Ambulatory Blood Pressure Monitoring (Fig. 3.5)

- 24-h BP: 129/69 mmHg; HR: 74 bpm
- Daytime BP: 132/73 mmHg; HR: 76 bpm
- Night-time BP: 123/59 mmHg; HR: 66 bpm

Prescriptions

✓ Periodical BP evaluation at home according to recommendations from current guidelines.
✓ Lifestyle recommendations are reinforced (regular physical activity and low caloric intake, increase fruit and vegetables, reduce sodium intake).

Which is the most useful diagnostic test to repeat during the follow-up in this patient in the next 6–12 months?

Possible answers are:

1. 24-h ambulatory BP monitoring
2. Echocardiogram
3. Vascular Doppler ultrasound
4. Chest X-rays

An echocardiogram could be particularly useful, together with an electrocardiogram. It has been shown that the regression of asymptomatic OD occurring during treatment is associated to a better prognosis, and the best demonstration of this concept has been obtained with electrocardiographic and echocardiographic indices of left ventricular hypertrophy [1].

3.5 Discussion

Cardiovascular diseases are among the leading causes of death worldwide. High BP is one of the most important risk factors for cardiovascular events and mortality. If left uncontrolled, hypertension predisposes to stroke and dementia, myocardial infarction, heart failure and renal insufficiency and imposes severe financial burdens on health systems [1, 3]. Despite clear evidence that BP-lowering strategies substantially reduce the risk, studies performed in several countries show that a noticeable proportion of hypertensive individuals are unaware of this condition or, if aware, are left untreated. Furthermore, in treated patients BP control is seldom obtained, in Europe and outside Europe [1, 3].

Among the possible mechanisms underlying the low rate of BP control, a relevant role seems to be played by physician inertia, by the insufficient adoption of correct lifestyle changes and by patient's low adherence and persistence to treatment [1, 5, 6]. It has been demonstrated that 6 months after starting antihypertensive treatment, more than one third of patients stop taking the drugs; at 1 year the proportion of patients stopping treatment further rises to 50 %. It has also been demonstrated that, even when antihypertensive treatment is not interrupted, adherence to the pharmacological plan (i.e. the extent to which the person's behaviour corresponds with agreed recommendations) is often only partial.

Investigating adherence to treatment, however, is very difficult, and in most cases physicians tend to overestimate patient's adherence to treatment.

This clinical case describes a patient who was seen at the hypertension clinic due to poor BP control despite treatment with three drugs at optimal dosage. The reason for referral was resistant hypertension. However, true resistant hypertension was ruled out: in fact in this case BP values begun to decrease soon after the first visit, probably due to a greater awareness of the patient of the risks associated to high BP and to an increased comprehension of the benefits associated with BP control.

The new therapeutic plan in this patient was based, firstly, on a better education.

Secondly, treatment strategy was simplified by using combination therapy, which is known to increase patient's adherence. In fact, it is well known that adherence to antihypertensive treatment decreases with increasing number of pills (Fig. 3.6) and that fixed dose combination therapy is an effective strategy for increasing patient's adherence [1]. A large meta-analysis on more than 30,000 patients has demonstrated that starting treatment with a fixed combination of drugs is associated with a significant improvement in adherence [8].

Some findings at the second visit seem also to indicate a change in the behaviour of the patient: heart rate fell significantly, possibly indicating the regular assumption of

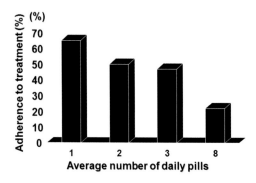

FIGURE 3.6 Adherence to treatment according to daily number of pills [7]

verapamil by the patient, and, in addition, BP values were not increased, and even mildly decreased, despite the initial reduction in the number of prescribed drugs.

In the subsequent visit further BP reduction was obtained by using a single-pill, fixed combination of an ACE inhibitor and a calcium channel blocker administered once daily.

A relevant aspect, possibly contributing to initial pseudo-resistance to treatment in this patient, is represented by lifestyle. In fact, factors such as high sodium intake or assumption of large amounts of alcohol should be carefully evaluated in patients with insufficient response to antihypertensive treatment. Prompt implementation of a correct lifestyle is crucial for the attainment of BP target.

Take-Home Messages

- Despite the clear evidence that BP reduction is associated to substantial benefits, BP control is inadequate in Europe and outside Europe.
- Uncontrolled hypertension does not mean "resistant" hypertension: pseudoresistance is not uncommon in everyday practice.
- Poor adherence to treatment is frequently responsible for inadequate BP control and should be sought carefully.
- Among the factors associated to poor adherence, the number of pills represents a crucial factor: as the number of pills increases, adherence to treatment decreases.
- Treatment strategies based on single-pill, fixed combinations of antihypertensive drugs are associated to better adherence to treatment and to improved BP control. For this reason current international Hypertension Guidelines favour the use of fixed combination.

References

1. Mancia G, Fagard R, Narkiewicz K, Redon J, Zanchetti A, Bohm M, et al. 2013 ESH/ESC Guidelines for the management of arterial hypertension: the Task Force for the management of arterial hypertension of the European Society of Hypertension (ESH) and of the European Society of Cardiology (ESC). J Hypertens. 2013;31(7):1281–357.
2. Reboldi G, Angeli F, Verdecchia P. Ambulatory blood pressure profile for risk stratification. Keep it simple. Hypertension. 2014; 63:913–4.
3. Global Burden of Metabolic Risk Factors for Chronic Diseases Collaboration. Cardiovascular disease, chronic kidney disease, and diabetes mortality burden of cardiometabolic risk factors from 1980 to 2010: a comparative risk assessment. Lancet Diabetes Endocrinol. 2014;2(8):634–47.
4. Tocci G, Ferrucci A, Pontremoli R, Ferri C, Agabiti Rosei E, Morganti A, Trimarco B, Mancia G, Borghi C, Volpe M. Blood pressure levels and control in Italy: comprehensive analysis of clinical data from 2000–2005 and 2005–2011 hypertension surveys. J Hum Hypertens. 2015;29(11):696–701.
5. Corrao G, Zambon A, Parodi A, Poluzzi E, Baldi I, Merlino L, et al. Discontinuation of and changes in drug therapy for hypertension among newly treated patients: a population-based study in Italy. J Hypertens. 2008;26(4):819–24.
6. Corrao G, Parodi A, Zambon A, Heiman F, Filippi A, Cricelli C, et al. Reduced discontinuation of antihypertensive treatment by two-drug combination as first step. Evidence from daily life practice. J Hypertens. 2010;28(7):1584–90.
7. Mancia G, Omboni S, Grassi G. Combination treatment in hypertension: the VeraTran Study. Am J Hypertens. 1997;10(7 Pt 2): 153S–8S.
8. Gupta AK, Arshad S, Poulter NR. Compliance, safety, and effectiveness of fixed-dose combinations of antihypertensive agents: a meta-analysis. Hypertension. 2010;55(2):399–407.

Clinical Case 4
Adult Patient with Pseudo-Resistant Hypertension: Drug Intolerance

4.1 Clinical Case Presentation

C. A., a 66-year-old Caucasian male, retired, former postman, was visited at the Hypertension Clinic as an outpatient for uncontrolled hypertension and mild leg oedema.

He had been diagnosed as having arterial hypertension when he was 50; at that time a complete workup for secondary hypertension had been performed, and a diagnosis of essential hypertension had been made. In particular renovascular hypertension, primary aldosteronism and Cushing disease and sleep apnoea had been excluded.

He is currently taking an ACE inhibitor/diuretic combination (enalapril 20 mg + hydrochlorothiazide 12.5 mg) in the morning and in the evening and an alpha-blocker, doxazosin, 4 mg OD in the evening.

The patient reports blood pressure readings above 150/90 mmHg at home. When he measures BP in the office of the general practitioner, values are constantly above 140/90 mmHg.

He declares to take regularly his antihypertensive treatment.

About 1 month ago, the patient was visited by the general practitioner for palpitations and poor home BP control. At the doctor's office, blood pressure values were 154/96 mmHg;

© Springer International Publishing Switzerland 2016   55
M. Salvetti, *Resistant Hypertension*, Practical
Case Studies in Hypertension Management,
DOI 10.1007/978-3-319-30637-7_4

treatment with enalapril + hydrochlorothiazide had been left unchanged, and doxazosin was increased from 2 mg OD to 4 mg OD, in the evening.

Family History

His father died at the age of 82 for colonic cancer; he was hypertensive and diabetic. His mother died at the age of 56 in a car crash; she was apparently healthy. He has one brother (60 years old), who is hypertensive. Also he has one sister (62 years), who is hypertensive. Another sister (58 years) is in good health.

He is married, he lives with his wife, and they have one son, who is in good health.

Clinical History

He smoked about 20 cigarettes per day until the age of 65. He drinks alcohol moderately (1–2 glasses of wine per day, no hard drinks) and has sedentary habits.

He is taking atorvastatin for hypercholesterolemia (20 mg once daily, in the evening).

He has also been diagnosed as having asthma, treated only with salbutamol in puffs in the very rare occasions of acute attacks.

About 5 years before, he had undergone left saphenectomy for symptomatic varicosities.

He is intolerant to calcium antagonists: about 10 years before the current visit, the general practitioner had introduced amlodipine 10 mg, but the drug had been stopped due to the appearance of leg oedema, which resolved after treatment cessation. A few years ago a new trial with a calcium antagonist (nifedipine slow release 60 mg) had been carried out, but the drug had been stopped due to symptomatic leg oedema.

There are no other known cardiovascular risk factor, associated clinical conditions or non-cardiovascular diseases.

Physical Examination

- Weight: 98 kg
- Height: 177 cm
- Body mass index (BMI): 31.3 kg/m^2
- Waist circumference: 106 cm
- Respiration: 13/min
- Heart: grade 1 systolic murmur at the apex
- Resting pulse: regular rhythm with normal heart rate (78 beats/min)
- Carotid arteries: no murmurs
- Femoral and foot arteries: palpable
- Clear lungs
- Mild lower extremity oedema
- Signs of venous insufficiency
- Remainder of the examination: normal

Haematological Profile

- Haemoglobin: 15.0 g/dL
- Haematocrit: 44 %
- Fasting plasma glucose: 99 mg/dL
- Fasting lipids: total cholesterol 186 mg/dL; HDL 43 mg/dL; triglycerides 145 mg/dL (LDL, Friedewald formula: 114 mg/dL)
- Electrolytes: sodium, 140 mEq/L; potassium, 4.1 mEq/L
- Serum uric acid: 5.4 mg/dL
- Renal function: creatinine, 1.0 mg/dL; estimated glomerular filtration rate (eGFR) (EPI formula: 78 mL/min/1.73 m^2)
- Urine analysis (dipstick): normal
- Urinary albumin excretion: not available
- Normal liver function tests
- TSH: not available

Blood Pressure Profile

Mr C. A. was measuring BP values at home with a wrist automatic device. He measures BP about two times per week, in supine position, in the evening after dinner (single measurement).

- Home BP was, on average, 160/95 mmHg, with wide variations (values from 110/60 to 180/108 mmHg).
- Office sitting BP: 164/102 mmHg; no difference between arms.
- Standing BP: 158/104 mmHg at 1 min.

  24-h BP monitoring had not been performed.

12-Lead Electrocardiogram

The electrocardiogram was substantially normal: sinus rhythm, absence of signs of left ventricular hypertrophy (Cornell voltage < 3.5 mV, Cornell product < 244 mV*ms, r aVL< 1.1 mV).

Normal repolarization, strain absent (Fig. 4.1).

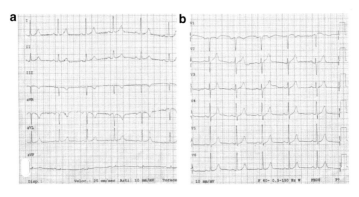

FIGURE 4.1 Electrocardiogram

The quality of sleep was investigated, daytime sleepiness was absent, the Epworth Sleepiness Scale score was evaluated, and sleep apnoea was judged unlikely.

Current Treatment

- ACE-i + diuretic fixed combination (enalapril 20 mg + hydrochlorothiazide 12.5 mg) at 8 am and at 8 pm
- Doxazosin mg OD, at 22 pm
- Atorvastatin 20 mg OD at 22 pm

Diagnosis

- **Essential hypertension, grade 2, with unsatisfactory BP control despite combination therapy with two drugs**
- **Intolerance to calcium antagonists (leg oedema)**
- **Asthma**
- Central obesity (grade 1, BMI 31)
- Hypercholesterolemia
- Sedentary habits
- No evidence of hypertension-related organ damage or associated clinical conditions

Which is the global cardiovascular risk profile in this patient?

Possible answers are:

1. Low
2. Moderate to high
3. High
4. Very high

Which is the best therapeutic option in this patient?
Possible answers are:

1. Add another drug, maintaining the other antihypertensives in use.
2. Change treatment.
3. Renal denervation.
4. Reinforce lifestyle changes.
5. 2+4.

Treatment Evaluation

✓ A full dose ACE inhibitor + full dose thiazide-like diuretic was added (single pill combination).
✓ Doxazosin was stopped (possible contributing to oedema).
✓ Lercanidipine low dose was added.
✓ Lifestyle measures were recommended.

Prescribed Treatment

– Perindopril 10 mg + indapamide 2.5 mg fixed combination once daily at 08.00 am
– Lercanidipine 10 mg once daily at 08.00 am
– Atorvastatin 20 mg OD at 22 pm

Prescriptions

✓ Lifestyle measures were recommended: the patient was instructed to increase physical activity (mild intensity, at least 4 days weekly) and to reduce caloric and salt intake.
✓ An echocardiogram, an ultrasound evaluation of the carotid arteries and assessment of albumin/creatinine ratio were prescribed, with the main aim of evaluating preclinical organ damage.

✓ Self BP measurement at home with an automated device (arm cuff). The use of wrist device was discouraged. Instructions for correct BP measurement were provided

✓ The patient was told that, despite the known intolerance to calcium antagonists, a short trial with a new-generation molecule could be worthwhile. Furthermore, it was not clear whether previous treatments with calcium antagonists had been in combination with renin angiotensin system (RAS) blockers, which are known to reduce the oedema induced by calcium antagonists. The patient was instructed to stop the calcium antagonist in case of evident symptomatic oedema and to go to the GP's office.

4.2 Follow-Up (Visit 1) at 6 Weeks

At follow-up visit, the patient was asymptomatic.

He had been taking the prescribed therapy for 1 week, but subsequently he had stopped lercanidipine due to symptomatic oedema.

He had measured blood pressure frequently, and mean home BP values were (on average) 140/85 mmHg.

He had only slightly improved his lifestyle by reducing salt intake and beginning to walk occasionally, and his weight was unchanged.

Physical Examination

- Weight: 98 kg
- Height: 177 cm
- Body mass index (BMI): 31.3 kg/m^2
- Waist circumference: 106 cm
- Resting pulse: regular rhythm with normal heart rate (76 beats/min)
- No oedema
- Other clinical parameters substantially unchanged

Blood Pressure Profile

- Home BP (average): 150/94 mmHg (mean of measure-ments in the morning and in the evening)
- Office sitting BP: 156/98 mmHg
- Standing BP: 152/98 mmHg at 1 min

Current Treatment

✓ Perindopril 10 mg + indapamide 2.5 mg fixed combination once daily at 08.00 am
✓ Atorvastatin 20 mg OD at 22 pm

Microalbuminuria

Albumin/creatinine ratio 19 mg/g

Echocardiogram

The echocardiogram showed normal left ventricular (LV) internal dimensions, thickness and mass (LV mass 160 g, LV mass index 34 g/m$^{2.7}$; relative wall thickness, 0.28) (Fig. 4.2). Systolic function was preserved (LV ejection fraction 55 %). The evaluation of Doppler indices of diastolic function with both conventional and tissue Doppler showed impaired LV relaxation (isovolumic relaxation time 107 msec), without signs of increased LV filling pressure (E/A ration 0.97, E dec time 190 msec, E/Em 9) (Fig. 4.3). Left atrial volume (23.3 ml/m^2) and the dimensions of the proximal aorta were normal. Mild mitral, aortic and tricuspid regurgitation were observed. Systolic pulmonary artery pressure is 28 mmHg. Inferior vena cava was not dilated.

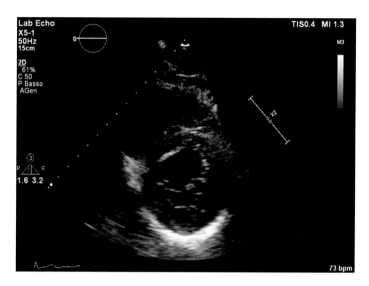

FIGURE 4.2 Echocardiogram: parasternal short axis view

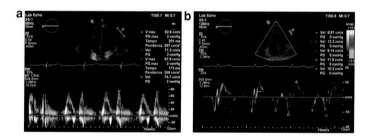

FIGURE 4.3 Echocardiogram: transmitral flow and tissue Doppler analysis

Ultrasound Evaluation of the Carotid Arteries (Fig. 4.4)

No evidence of stenosis.

There are plaques, with regular surface and maximum thickness 1.7 mm, at the bifurcations of the carotid arteries, bilaterally.

Vertebral arteries: normal flow.

Which is the global cardiovascular risk profile in this patient after further assessment of organ damage?

Possible answers are:

1. Low
2. Moderate to high
3. High
4. Very high

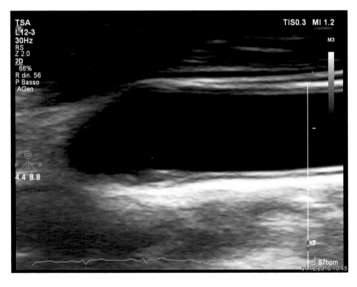

FIGURE 4.4 Carotid ultrasound

According to ESH ESC 2013 Guidelines, CV risk is at least high in this patient. In fact, a large amount of data indicate that the presence of carotid plaques identifies patients at high CV risk [1, 2] (Fig. 4.5).

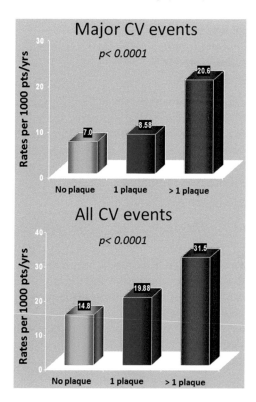

FIGURE 4.5 Incidence of cardiovascular events according to the presence of carotid plaques in ELSA study

Diagnosis

A diagnosis was made:

- Essential hypertension, grade 2, with unsatisfactory BP control due to drug intolerance
- Vascular preclinical organ damage (small carotid plaque)
- Intolerance to calcium antagonists (leg oedema)
- Intolerance to doxazosin (mild leg oedema)

– **Bronchial asthma**
– **Central obesity (grade 1, BMI 31)**
– **Hypercholesterolemia**
– **Sedentary habits**

Treatment with a new-generation dihydropyridine, despite being usually better tolerated as compared to first-generation molecules, was unsuccessful in this patient: in fact leg oedema rapidly appeared. Therefore, drug intolerance, together with the presence of comorbidities (asthma), limits substantially the choice of drugs in this patient

Treatment Evaluation

✓ Treatment with the ACE-i/diuretic was maintained.
✓ 24-h ambulatory blood pressure monitoring after 4 weeks was scheduled, in order to confirm inadequate BP control despite changes lifestyle.
✓ Doxazosin was not restarted, since the patient had noted mild oedema when taking the alpha-blocker (oedema has now completely disappeared).

Prescribed Treatment

– Perindopril 10 mg + indapamide 2.5 mg fixed combination once daily at 08.00 am

Prescriptions

✓ Periodical BP evaluation at home according to recommendations from current guidelines
✓ Regular physical activity and low caloric and salt intake. Diet rich in fruits and vegetables
✓ Assays for plasma creatinine, sodium and potassium before the next visit (possible addition of antialdosterone agent in case of uncontrolled BP)

4.3   Follow-Up (Visit 2) After Further 4 Weeks

At follow-up visit, the patient was fine.

He started following a healthier lifestyle. He has reduced calories and fat intake and regular mild physical activity, three times per week. His weight is slightly improved (– 3 kg in 6 weeks).

Physical Examination

- Weight: 95 kg
- Height: 177 cm
- Body mass index (BMI): 30.3 kg/m^2
- Waist circumference: 104 cm
- Resting pulse: regular rhythm with 72 beats/min
- Other parameters substantially unchanged

Blood Pressure Profile

- Home BP (average): 144/88 mmHg (early morning)
- Sitting BP: 150/100 mmHg (mean of three measurements, in sitting position)
- Standing BP: 146/90 mmHg

Ambulatory Blood Pressure Monitoring

- 24-h BP: 138/96 mmHg; HR: 74 bpm.
- Daytime BP: 138/99 mmHg; HR: 77 bpm.
- Night-time BP: 139/88 mmHg; HR: 70 bpm.
- There was no reduction of systolic BP values during the night. Blood pressure variability was not increased (standard deviation of night-time SBP 8.9 mmHg).

The 24-h ambulatory blood pressure profile is illustrated in Fig. 4.6.

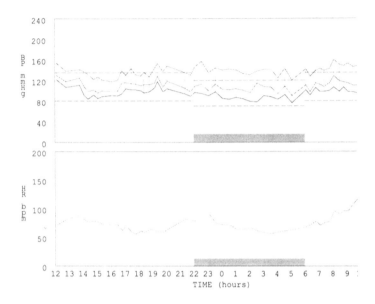

FIGURE 4.6 24-hour blood pressure profile at second follow-up visit

Renal Function Parameters

- Creatinine, 1.1 mg/dL; estimated glomerular filtration rate (eGFR) (EPI formula: 70 mL/min/1.73 m^2)
- Electrolytes: sodium, 141 mEq/L; potassium, 4.0 mEq/L

Current Treatment

- Perindopril 10 mg + indapamide 2.5 mg fixed combination once daily at 08.00 am
- Atorvastatin 20 mg OD at 22 pm

Treatment Evaluation

✓ A mineralocorticoid receptor antagonist at low dose was added.
✓ The combination of ACEI and diuretic was maintained.

Treatment prescribed

✓ Perindopril 10 mg + indapamide 2.5 mg fixed combination once daily at 08.00 am
✓ Canrenone 25 mg once daily at 08.00 am

Prescriptions

✓ Control of creatinine, sodium and potassium at 3 and 8 weeks (use of potassium sparing diuretic) and frequently thereafter
✓ Home BP measurement according to recommendations from current guidelines
✓ Regular follow-up visits at the office of the general practitioner (if BP not well controlled further evaluation at the Hypertension Clinic, after at least 6 weeks of treatment and lifestyle changes)

4.4   Follow-Up (Visit 3) at 3 Months

The patient came to the Hypertension Clinic for a follow-up visit.

He had regularly measured BP with an automated, validated arm device.

He had also been visited repeatedly by the family doctor.

He was in good clinical conditions, and his lifestyle was improved: he was performing mild intensity physical activity 3–4 times per week and was trying to limit salt, calories and fat foods, increasing vegetables and fruit.

Physical Examination

• Weight: 91 kg
• Body mass index (BMI): 29.1 kg/m^2
• Waist circumference: 99 cm
• Resting pulse: regular rhythm with 66 beats/min
• No leg oedema
• Other parameters substantially unchanged

Blood Pressure Profile

- Home BP (average): 136/84 mmHg
- Sitting BP: 140/90 mmHg
- Standing BP: 138/92 mmHg

Renal Function Parameters

- Creatinine, 1.1 mg/dL; estimated glomerular filtration rate (eGFR) (EPI formula: 70 mL/min/1.73 m^2)
- Electrolytes: sodium, 140 mEq/L; potassium, 4.5 mEq/L

12-Lead Electrocardiogram

The electrocardiogram was substantially unchanged, showing sinus rhythm and no ST-segment abnormalities or signs of LVH.

Current Treatment

✓ Perindopril 10 mg + indapamide 2.5 mg fixed combination once daily at 08.00 am
✓ Canrenone 25 mg once daily at 08.00 am
✓ Atorvastatin 20 mg OD at 22 pm

Treatment Evaluation

✓ No changes for current pharmacological therapy

Prescriptions

✓ The main objective for this patient will be to further improve lifestyle, trying to further reduce calories and salt intake and to increase physical activity.

✓ Periodical BP evaluation at home according to recommendations from current guidelines.

✓ Control of creatinine, sodium and potassium at regular intervals (interval of about 2–3 months).

4.5 Discussion

Appropriate management of patients with arterial hypertension represents one of the main objectives for cardiovascular disease prevention. Despite the increasing awareness of the dramatic consequences of high BP, in a large proportion of patients, BP targets are not achieved.

This clinical case well describes the difficulties in reaching BP target in everyday practice. In fact, in some patients, the armamentarium available for the treatment of hypertension is not so well stocked with drugs. Indeed, drug intolerance is not uncommon. The use of calcium antagonists, which are among the most effective antihypertensive drugs, is often limited by the occurrence of leg oedema. The mechanism underlying this side effect is related to a decrease in arteriolar resistance, which leads to a change in hydrostatic pressures in the precapillary circulation, thereby increasing fluid exudation from the intracapillary space into the interstitium. The occurrence of leg oedema is more frequent in women and with increasing age, possibly due to the protective effect of the greater elasticity of the skin and subcutaneous tissue in younger patients; warm conditions may contribute to worsen oedema. Calcium antagonist-related oedema is dose dependent; however, it has been demonstrated that at equipotent doses, it is much less evident with new-generation dihydropyridines, such as lercanidipine, barnidipine lacidipine or manidipine [2–4]. For this reason, in this patient a short trial of a new-generation calcium antagonist was made. The calcium channel blocker was combined with an ACE inhibitor: this may exert favourable effects on calcium channel blocker-related oedema, which is much less frequent when calcium antagonists are combined with ACE inhibitors or angiotensin receptor blockers, possibly due to the vasodilating properties of these drugs [3, 4]. Of note, the favourable effect of RAS blockers on this type of oedema is superior to that of diuretics [4].

The patient described in this clinical case did not tolerate the new-generation calcium antagonist, even in combination with an ACE inhibitor and a diuretic. In these cases the only option is represented by the discontinuation of the drug. Therefore, it was not possible to take advantage of the synergistic effect of a calcium channel blocker with a RAS blocker and a diuretic. This combination probably represents the most effective and well-studied combination of three drugs for the treatment of hypertension. The presence of asthma further limited the choice of drugs. In fact, asthma represents one of the few absolute contraindications to beta blockers [2]. Furthermore, it was also necessary to discontinue doxazosin, due to oedema, a possible side effect of alpha-blockers [5]. Therefore, another drug with demonstrated antihypertensive efficacy could not be used in this patient.

Therefore, the choice of the third drug was made empirically. Mineralocorticoid receptor antagonists are not among the recommended first-line drugs for hypertension, due to the limited data from randomized clinical trials available but, as also indicated by the ESH ESC Hypertension Guidelines, can be used as a third- or fourth-line drugs, being among the most effective additional antihypertensive drugs, provided the possible adverse effects on renal function are adequately monitored [2, 6, 7]. When using mineralocorticoid receptor antagonists in hypertensive patients, the use of low doses is advisable, in order to minimize possible side effects such as gynecomastia, impotence or diminished libido in males or menstrual alterations and breast tenderness in female patients.

Take-Home Messages

- Drug intolerance is relatively common and may represent an obstacle to the achievement of BP target in hypertensive patients.
- Among the most common side effects of antihypertensive drugs are peripheral oedema, cough, bronchoconstriction, metabolic disturbances, AV block, angioedema and hormonal alterations.
- Peripheral oedema is relatively frequent in patients treated with calcium antagonists, which are among the most effective antihypertensive drugs and particularly effective in combination treatment. The mechanism underlying this side effect is related to a decrease in arteriolar resistance and to a change in hydrostatic pressures in the precapillary circulation, leading to fluid exudation into the interstitium.
- Also other drug classes may favour peripheral oedema: the alpha-blockers or the less frequently used direct arteriolar dilators minoxidil and hydralazine.
- Tailoring treatment to the patient's characteristics is particularly important when drug intolerance is present, since it may allow the attainment of blood pressure targets.

References

1. Zanchetti A, Bond MG, Hennig M, Neiss A, Mancia G, Dal Palù C, Hansson L, Magnani B, Rahn KH, Reid JL, Rodicio J, Safar M, Eckes L, Rizzini P, European Lacidipine Study on Atherosclerosis investigators. Calcium antagonist lacidipine slows down progression of asymptomatic carotid atherosclerosis: principal results of the European Lacidipine Study on Atherosclerosis (ELSA), a randomized, double-blind, long-term trial. Circulation. 2002; 106(19):2422–7.

2. Mancia G, Fagard R, Narkiewicz K, Redon J, Zanchetti A, Bohm M, et al. 2013 ESH/ESC Guidelines for the management of arterial hypertension: the Task Force for the management of arterial hypertension of the European Society of Hypertension (ESH) and of the European Society of Cardiology (ESC). J Hypertens. 2013;31(7):1281–357.
3. De la Sierra A. Mitigation of calcium channel blocker-related oedema in hypertension by antagonists of the renin-angiotensin system. J Hum Hypertens. 2009;23(8):503–11.
4. Messerli FH. Vasodilatory edema: a common side effect of anti-hypertensive therapy. Curr Cardiol Rep. 2002;4(6):479–82.
5. Chapman N, Chang CL, Dahlöf B, Sever PS, Wedel H, Poulter NR, ASCOT Investigators. Effect of doxazosin gastrointestinal therapeutic system as third-line antihypertensive therapy on blood pressure and lipids in the Anglo-Scandinavian Cardiac Outcomes Trial. Circulation. 2008;118(1):42–8.
6. Chapman N, Dobson J, Wilson S, et al. Effect of spironolactone on blood pressure in subjects with resistant hypertension. Hypertension. 2007;49:839–45.
7. Williams B, MacDonald TM, Morant S, Webb DJ, Sever P, McInnes G, Ford I, Cruickshank JK, Caulfield MJ, Salsbury J, Mackenzie I, Padmanabhan S, Brown MJ, British Hypertension Society's PATHWAY Studies Group. Spironolactone versus placebo, bisoprolol, and doxazosin to determine the optimal treatment for drug-resistant hypertension (PATHWAY-2): a randomised, double-blind, crossover trial. Lancet. 2015;386: 2059–68.

Clinical Case 5

Adult Patient with Pseudo-Resistant Hypertension: Spurious Resistant Hypertension

5.1 Clinical Case Presentation

M. G., a 60-year-old Caucasian female, retired saleswoman, was seen at the Hypertension Clinic for a visit.

She came to the office because, despite combination anti-hypertensive therapy, blood pressure values remained elevated in most occasions.

She was substantially asymptomatic, with the exception of mild palpitations, only at rest.

Family History

Her mother, 92 years old, was hypertensive and had type 2 diabetes mellitus. Her father died at the age of 78 for septic shock; he had Alzheimer's disease since he was 72 years old. She had one brother and one sister (65 and 62 years old, respectively), both treated for arterial hypertension. They were both dyslipidemic. She was single and lived with her mother and her sister.

© Springer International Publishing Switzerland 2016
M. Salvetti, *Resistant Hypertension*, Practical
Case Studies in Hypertension Management,
DOI 10.1007/978-3-319-30637-7_5

Clinical History

She was a current smoker (she had smoked about 20 cigarettes per day between the ages of 16 and 50; when she was 60 she had reduced the number of cigarettes to about 10 per day). She did not drink alcohols.

She was sedentary, and her diet was rich in vegetables; salt intake was not low.

Arterial hypertension had been diagnosed when she was 52 years old, about 1 year after menopause. She had been at the office of the general practitioner because BP values recorded with the automated wrist device of her mother were elevated.

The general practitioner had recorded values in the grade 2 range and, after a period of about 2 months of observation with lifestyle measures, had started treatment with transdermal clonidine.

After a period of years of good BP control, about 3 years before the visit, BP values had progressively increased, and the general practitioner had added candesartan, initially at the dosage of 16 mg OD and, after a few weeks, 32 mg OD.

An abdominal ultrasound scan performed 1 year before the visit for transient abdominal pain was substantially normal.

Comorbidities

– Duodenal ulcer (diagnosed in 2005; *Helicobacter pylori* had been eradicated and after that she had been asymptomatic).
– Surgery for inguinal hernia in 2002.
– Gilbert's syndrome.
– Some years before depression had been diagnosed. After a period of treatment with antidepressants, her mood had improved and treatment had been stopped.

There are no other known cardiovascular risk factors, associated clinical conditions or non-cardiovascular diseases.

Physical Examination

- Weight: 74 kg
- Height: 162 cm
- Body mass index (BMI): 28.2 kg/m^2
- Waist circumference: 86 cm
- Respiration: 12/min
- Heart sounds: S1–S2 regular, no murmurs
- Resting pulse: regular rhythm, 72 beats/min
- Carotid arteries: no murmurs
- Femoral and foot arteries: palpable
- Clear lungs
- No lower extremity oedema
- Remainder of the examination: normal

Haematological Profile

- Haemoglobin: 12.9 g/dL
- Mean corpuscular volume: 85
- WBC $6.7 \times 10^3/\mu L$
- PLT $325 \times 10^3/\mu L$
- Fasting plasma glucose: 88 mg/dL
- Fasting lipids: total cholesterol 200 mg/dL, HDL 82 mg/dL, LDL 95 mg/dL, triglycerides 113 mg/dL
- Electrolytes: sodium, 141 mEq/L; potassium, 4.6 mEq/L
- Serum uric acid: 5.0 mg/dL
- Renal function: creatinine 0.85 mg/dL, eGFR CKD-EPI 74 mL/min/1.73 m^2
- Urine analysis (dipstick): normal
- Albuminuria: albumin/creatinine ratio: not available
- Liver function tests normal
- TSH: not tested

Blood Pressure Profile

Mr. M. G. does measure blood pressure at home (1–2 measurements per week, with a wrist automated device).

The available measurements show values ranging from 140 to 165 mmHg for systolic and from 85 to 100 for diastolic.

BP measurements during the visit:

- Office sitting BP: 156/90 mmHg; no difference between the two arms
- Standing BP: 144/90 mmHg at 1 min
- Ambulatory blood pressure monitoring: not available

12-Lead Electrocardiogram

The electrocardiogram showed sinus rhythm, no evidence of left ventricular hypertrophy and normal repolarization (Fig. 5.1).

Current Treatment

– Transdermal clonidine (TTS 1, 2.5 mg) 1 application/week
– Candesartan 32 mg 1 cp once daily (h 08.00)

Which is the global cardiovascular risk profile in this patient?

Possible answers are:

1. Low
2. Moderate
3. High
4. Very high

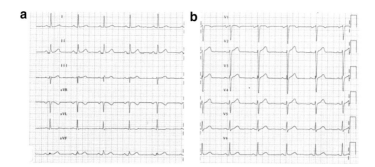

FIGURE 5.1 (**a**, **b**) Electrocardiogram

Global Cardiovascular Risk Stratification

According to 2013 ESH/ESC global cardiovascular risk stratification [1], this patient has a moderate cardiovascular risk profile (grade 1 arterial hypertension with 1 additional CV risk factor).

Workup

The strong family history for hypertension and the moderate elevation of BP suggest an essential hypertension. An echo-cardiogram was prescribed for a better evaluation of organ damage.

Treatment Evaluation

✓ Clonidine was withdrawn. In fact the drug is not among the first-line drugs for hypertension treatment according to current guideline [1], and furthermore, due to the possible effect on depressive symptoms, it is not an ideal option for this patient.

✓ Candesartan was maintained, but was administered as fixed-dose combination with hydrochlorothiazide. Nifedipine chrono was also added.

Treatment Prescribed

– Candesartan 32 mg/hydrochlorothiazide 25 mg 1 cp once daily (h 08.00)
– Nifedipine chrono 30 mg once daily (h 08.00)

Prescriptions

✓ Lifestyle changes were recommended, in particular low-salt diet, rich in fruit and vegetables and regular moderate physical activity.
✓ Adherence to treatment was recommended.
✓ The patient was instructed to measure BP at home with a standardized approach (sitting for at least 5 min in a quiet room, repeating measurements 2–3 times in each occasion and recording the mean value).
✓ An echocardiogram and an Holter ECG (palpitations) were also prescribed.

5.2   Follow-Up (Visit 1) at 6 Weeks

At follow-up visit, the patient was asymptomatic.

She had increased the number of measurements of blood pressure. Mean values at home were still elevated and highly variable.

Body weight was unchanged.

The patient declared to be adherent to antihypertensive treatment.

No drug-related side effects were reported.

Physical Examination

• Weight: 74 kg
• Height: 162 cm
• Body mass index (BMI): 28.2 kg/m^2

- Resting pulse: regular rhythm with normal heart rate (76 beats/min)
- Other clinical parameters substantially unchanged

Blood Pressure Profile

- Office sitting BP: 150/88 mmHg
- Standing BP: 146/90 mmHg at 1 min

Current Treatment

– Candesartan 32 mg/hydrochlorothiazide 25 mg 1 cp once daily (h 08.00)
– Nifedipine chrono 30 mg once daily (h 08.00)

Haematological Profile

- Albuminuria: albumin/creatinine ratio, 12 mg/g

Echocardiogram

The echocardiogram showed normal LV internal dimensions, mass and geometry (LVMI 35 g/m$^{2.7}$, RWT 0.27) (Fig. 5.2), with preserved systolic function. Left atrial diameter and volume were normal (volume 25 mL/BSA). LV diastolic parameters were normal; TDI: E/E^1 6.2.

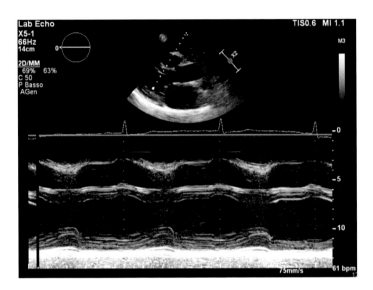

FIGURE 5.2 Echocardiogram

Carotid-Femoral Pulse Wave Velocity

Pulse wave velocity was normal: 8 m/s (cut-off for organ damage according to ESH/ESC Hypertension Guidelines >10 m/s).

Holter ECG

Constant sinus rhythm; occasional supraventricular premature beats (in one occasion corresponding to reported palpitations on the patient's diary). Normal findings.

Treatment Evaluation

   ✓ Treatment with a combination of three drugs was maintained, and the dosage of the calcium antagonist was increased.

Treatment Prescribed

- Candesartan 32 mg/hydrochlorothiazide 25 mg 1 cp once daily (h 08.00)
- Nifedipine chrono 60 mg once daily (h 08.00)

Prescriptions

✓ Regular physical activity and low caloric intake were recommended.
✓ Periodical BP evaluation at home at the upper arms according to recommendations from current guidelines.
✓ Adherence to treatment was recommended.

5.3   Follow-Up (Visit 2) at 12 Weeks

At follow-up visit at 12 weeks, the patient was well and asymptomatic.
   She had further improved her lifestyle.
   Her weight, however, was unchanged.
   Self-reported adherence to treatment was good.
   No drug-related side effects were reported.

Physical Examination

- Weight: 74 kg
- Height: 162 cm
- Body mass index (BMI): 28.2 kg/m^2
- Resting pulse: regular rhythm with normal heart rate (76 beats/min)
- Other clinical parameters substantially unchanged

Current Treatment

- Candesartan 32 mg/hydrochlorothiazide 25 mg 1 cp once daily (h 08.00)
- Nifedipine chrono 60 mg once daily (h 08.00)

Blood Pressure Profile

- Office sitting BP: 144/82 mmHg
- Standing BP: 142/88 mmHg at 1 min
- Home BP (average): 134/82 mmHg

The ambulatory blood pressure monitoring profile showed 24 h BP values below the thresholds, both during the day and the night, indicating achievement of adequate BP control with the current treatment.

- 24-h BP: 120/78 mmHg; HR: 62 bpm
- Daytime BP: 125/82 mmHg; HR: 66 bpm
- Night-time BP: 112/71 mmHg; HR: 54 bpm

The analysis of 24-h blood pressure profile shows increased BP variability during daytime, but BP variability was not increased during the night (standard deviation of night-time SBP: 8.15).

Day-to-night BP reduction was 10.5 %.

Figure 5.3 shows the 24-h ambulatory blood pressure profile.

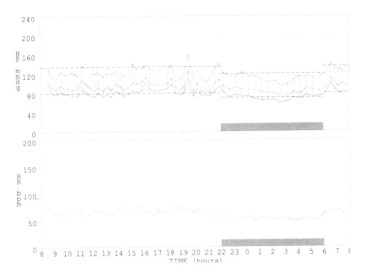

FIGURE 5.3 24-hour blood pressure profile

Current Treatment

– Candesartan 32 mg/hydrochlorothiazide 25 mg 1 cp once daily (h 08.00)
– Nifedipine chrono 60 mg once daily (h 08.00)

Treatment Evaluation

✓ The combination of an ARB; a diuretic and a calcium antagonist was maintained.

Treatment Prescribed

– Candesartan 32 mg/hydrochlorothiazide 25 mg 1 cp once daily (h 08.00)
– Nifedipine chrono 60 mg once daily (h 08.00)

Prescriptions

✓ The patient was instructed to continue to improve her lifestyle and to quit smoking.
✓ Home BP measurement was recommended, together with periodic BP measurement at the office of the general practitioner.

5.4   Follow-Up (Visit 3) at 6 Months

The patient was seen at the Hypertension Clinic for a control visit.
She was asymptomatic.
Her lifestyle was discretely improved.
Her weight was slightly reduced.
She was continuing moderate physical activity.

Physical Examination

- Weight: 71 kg
- Height: 162 cm
- Body mass index (BMI): 27.05 kg/m^2
- Resting pulse: regular rhythm with normal heart rate (72 beats/min)

Blood Pressure Profile

- Office sitting BP: 144/84 mmHg
- Standing BP: 138/88 mmHg at 1 min
- Home BP (average): 132/82 mmHg

Current Treatment

- Candesartan 32 mg/hydrochlorothiazide 25 mg 1 cp once daily (h 08.00)
- Nifedipine chrono 60 mg once daily (h 08.00)

Treatment Evaluation

✓ The combination of ARB/diuretic + calcium antagonist was left unchanged.

Treatment Prescribed

- Candesartan 32 mg/hydrochlorothiazide 25 mg 1 cp once daily (h 08.00)
- Nifedipine chrono 60 mg once daily (h 08.00)

Prescriptions

✓ Lifestyle recommendations were reinforced (regular physical activity and low caloric intake, increase fruit and vegetables, reduce sodium intake).
✓ BP measurements at home were recommended.

5.5   Discussion

This clinical case describes a patient with uncontrolled hypertension. This is quite common, since available data indicate that the majority of patients do not reach appropriate BP values despite treatment. In the EURIKA study, which included in 2009 7641 outpatients from 12 European countries, aged ≥50 years and free of clinical CVD, among treated hypertensives (94.2 % of the total), only 38.8 % achieved the blood pressure target (Fig. 5.4).

In this patient the initial combination of drugs was not optimal: clonidine is not among the first-line drugs recommended by guidelines for hypertension [2], and furthermore, depression represents a contraindication for this drug. Despite an appropriate change in treatment regimen in the following

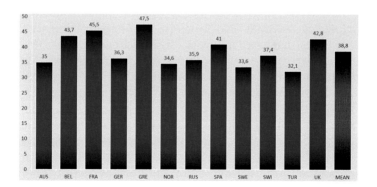

FIGURE 5.4 Achievement of blood pressure goal in Europe among treated patients, by country. Data from [1]

visits (ARB + diuretic and, subsequently, also a calcium antagonist), the BP target (<140/90 mmHg) was apparently not reached.

When patients fail to reach the BP target, a crucial aspect of the evaluation is represented by the confirmation of a true persistent elevation of BP values despite treatment.

In fact, a more accurate evaluation of BP values may allow the identification of a subset of patients with false resistant hypertension [2, 3]. The considerable variability of BP values at home reported by this patient might indicate that BP measurements were not properly done. In everyday clinical practice, hypertensive patients are worried by elevated BP values which are very often the result of inadequate knowledge of the methodology for BP measurement. Therefore, physicians should explain during the visit the correct technique for self-BP measurement (and verify the use of validated devices, properly calibrated). In addition to this, when resistant hypertension is suspected, ambulatory BP monitoring represents an important part of the workup, allowing the confirmation of true resistance to treatment. In the Spanish Ambulatory Blood Pressure Monitoring Registry [4], which included about 70,000 treated hypertensive patients, 12 % had resistant hypertension, defined as office BP ≥140 mmHg and/or 90 mmHg while on ≥3 antihypertensive drugs. In this study, after ABPM, only about two thirds of patients initially defined as "resistant" had "true resistant" hypertension, with 38 % being diagnosed as having "white-coat resistance". This study, as well as several other studies [5], has also shown that patients with true resistant hypertension have a higher prevalence of electrocardiographic and echocardiographic left ventricular hypertrophy, as well as of vascular and renal damage, which may explain the increase in CV risk in these patients but may also render hypertension more difficult to control. The absence of organ damage in patients referred for resistant hypertension should raise the suspect of "false resistance" and prompt the execution of ABPM (home BP measurement may be an alternative if BP is properly measured, with an automated and validated device) [2]. Interestingly, the finding of controlled 24 h BP values (also called "false" or "spurious" or "white-coat" resistant hypertension) is associated to a better prognosis [6–8]. For this reason, ABPM should be always performed before a diagnosis of resistant hypertension is made [9].

Take-Home Messages

- About **one third** of patients referred for **resistant hypertension have BP values well controlled at ABPM.**
- Treated patients with uncontrolled "office" BP but controlled "out-of-office" BP (24 h or home BP) have been defined as having **"spurious" or "false" or "white-coat" resistant hypertension.**
- Several studies have demonstrated that **"spurious"** (or "white-coat") **resistant hypertension is associated to a better prognosis** as compared to "true" resistant hypertension.
- **Confirmation of elevated BP by ABPM in all patients is advisable** before a diagnosis of resistant hypertension is made.

References

1. Banegas J, Lopez-Garcı E, Dallongeville J, Guallar E, Halcox J, Borghi C, Masso Gonzalez E, Jimenez F, Perk J, Steg P, De Backer G, Rodrıguez-Artalejo F. Achievement of treatment goals for primary prevention of cardiovascular disease in clinical practice across Europe: the EURIKA study.
2. Mancia G, Fagard R, Narkiewicz K, Redon J, Zanchetti A, Bohm M, et al. 2013 ESH/ESC Guidelines for the management of arterial hypertension: the Task Force for the management of arterial hypertension of the European Society of Hypertension (ESH) and of the European Society of Cardiology (ESC). J Hypertens. 2013;31(7):1281–357.

3. Calhoun D, Booth J, Oparil S, Irvin M, Shimbo D, Lackland D, Howard G, Safford M, Muntner P. Refractory hypertension determination of prevalence, risk factors, and comorbidities in a large, population-based cohort. Hypertension. 2014;63:451–8.
4. De la Sierra A, Segura J, Banegas JR, et al. Clinical features of 8295 patients with resistant hypertension classified on the basis of ambulatory blood pressure monitoring. Hypertension. 2011;57: 898e902.
5. Muiesan ML, Salvetti M, Rizzoni D, Paini A, Agabiti-Rosei C, Aggiusti C, Agabiti RE. Resistant hypertension and target organ damage. Hypertens Res. 2013;36(6):485–91.
6. Salles G, Cardoso C, Muxfeldt E. Prognostic influence of office and ambulatory blood pressures in resistant hypertension. Arch Intern Med. 2008;168:2340–6.
7. Muxfeldt ES, Cardoso CRL, Salles G. Prognostic value of the nocturnal blood pressure reduction in resistant hypertension. Arch Intern Med. 2009;169:874–80.
8. Pierdomenico SD, Lapenna D, Bucci A, Di Tommaso R, Di Mascio R, Manente BM, Caldarella MP, Neri M, Cuccurullo F, Mezzetti A. Cardiovascular outcome in treated hypertensive patients with responder, masked, false resistant, and true resistant hypertension. Am J Hypertens. 2005;18:1422–8.
9. Persu A, O'Brien E, Verdecchia P. Use of ambulatory blood pressure measurement in the definition of resistant hypertension: a review of the evidence. Hypertens Res. 2014;37(11):967–72.

Clinical Case 6

Adult Patient with Resistant Hypertension Secondary to Comorbidities

6.1 Clinical Case Presentation

D. M., a 67-year-old Caucasian male, farmer, was seen at the Hypertension Clinic for a visit.

He was referred by his general practitioner since blood pressure (BP) values were elevated despite antihypertensive treatment with three drugs: an ACE inhibitor, a thiazide diuretic and a beta blocker.

He reported mild reduction of exercise tolerance, but a recent treadmill exercise test was within limits.

Family History

His mother, 89 years old, was hypertensive and had permanent atrial fibrillation. His father died at the age of 72 due to gastric cancer and was hypertensive. He had one sister (65 years old) on treatment with statins for hypercholesterolemia. He lived with his wife, who was in good health, and they had one healthy daughter.

© Springer International Publishing Switzerland 2016   91
M. Salvetti, *Resistant Hypertension*, Practical
Case Studies in Hypertension Management,
DOI 10.1007/978-3-319-30637-7_6

Clinical History

He was a former smoker (at least 10 cigarettes per day between the ages of 17 and 55). He drunk alcoholics (he declared to drink about 1 L of wine every day and, "occasionally", hard drinks).

He was sedentary, and his diet was rich in meat and salt, poor in vegetables.

He had been overweight since when he had been a child, and his body weight tended to increase slightly till the age of 35; after that age, weight gain had been faster, constantly throughout years.

Arterial hypertension was diagnosed when he was 50 years old. At that time he had been visited at the office of the general practitioner because of an episode of acute bronchitis; BP had been measured, and grade 3 arterial hypertension had been diagnosed. He had been unable to report previous BP values ("…I have never measured BP…"), but further BP measurements had confirmed the diagnosis of grade 3 hypertension.

A workup for secondary hypertension was undertaken. No evident cause of endocrine hypertension was detected. An abdominal ultrasound scan and an echo colour Doppler examination of the renal arteries were substantially normal. Treatment with an ACE inhibitor was started. After some months a beta blocker was added.

About 8 months ago, a diuretic was added, since BP control was inadequate.

Comorbidities

– Reflux oesophagitis (diagnosed in 2009)
– Laparoscopic cholecystectomy

There are no other known cardiovascular risk factors, associated clinical conditions or non-cardiovascular diseases.

Physical Examination

- Weight: 110 kg
- Height: 175 cm
- Body mass index (BMI): 36 kg/m^2
- Waist circumference: 120 cm
- Respiration: 12/min
- Heart sounds: S1–S2 regular, no murmurs
- Resting pulse: regular rhythm, 66 beats/min
- Carotid arteries: no murmurs
- Femoral and foot arteries: palpable
- Clear lungs
- No lower extremity oedema
- Remainder of the examination: normal

Haematological Profile

- Haemoglobin: 14.4 g/dL
- Mean corpuscular volume: 88
- WBC $7.5 \times 10^3/\mu L$
- PLT $310 \times 10^3/\mu L$
- Fasting plasma glucose: 112 mg/dL
- Fasting lipids: total cholesterol 240 mg/dL, HDL 42 mg/dL, LDL 170 mg/dL, triglycerides 140 mg/dL
- Electrolytes: sodium, 140 mEq/L; potassium, 4.8 mEq/L
- Serum uric acid: 6.0 mg/dL
- Renal function: creatinine 1.25 mg/dL, eGFR CKD-EPI 59 mL/min/1.73 m^2
- Urine analysis (dipstick): unremarkable
- Albuminuria: albumin/creatinine ratio, not available (available one performed in 2011: ACR = 20 mg/g)
- Liver function tests normal
- TSH: not tested

Blood Pressure Profile

Mr. D.M. does not measure regularly blood pressure at home.
   However, the few available measurements indicate poor
blood pressure control: values are highly variable, but almost
always over the suggested cut-offs, ranging from 145 to
170 mmHg for systolic and from 75 to 85 for diastolic.

- Office sitting BP: 172/82 mmHg; no difference between the
  two arms. Heart rate 66 r
- Standing BP: 164/90 mmHg at 1 min
- Ambulatory blood pressure monitoring: not available

12-Lead Electrocardiogram

An electrocardiogram performed some months before the
visit showed sinus rhythm and no evidence of left ventricular
hypertrophy (Fig. 6.1).

Vascular Ultrasound

Echo Doppler evaluation of the carotid arteries showed
small plaques with regular surface at the level of the carotid
bifurcations and of the internal carotid arteries (Fig. 6.2a, b).

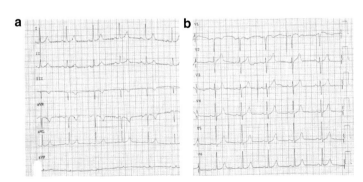

FIGURE 6.1 (**a**, **b**) Electrocardiogram

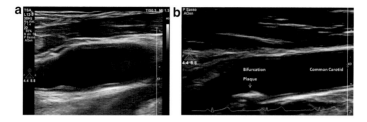

FIGURE 6.2 (**a, b**) Ultrasound scan of the carotid arteries

There is normal flow in the vertebral arteries.

As previously reported, screening for secondary hypertension and for specific causes of chronic kidney disease had been performed at the time of the diagnosis of arterial hypertension.

A new abdominal ultrasound performed about 5 years before for transient abdominal pain was substantially normal.

Once more, during the visit the possible presence of sleep apnoea was evaluated, involving also the patient's wife in the interview. The STOP-Bang Questionnaire score was intermediate (=4).

Current Treatment

– Ramipril 10 mg once daily (h 08.00)
– Atenolol 100 mg once daily (h 08.00) (dosage recently increased)
– Hydrochlorothiazide 25 mg (h 8.00)

Which is the global cardiovascular risk profile in this patient?

Possible answers are:

1. Low
2. Medium
3. High
4. Very high

Global Cardiovascular Risk Stratification

According to 2013 ESH/ESC global cardiovascular risk stratification [1], this patient has a high cardiovascular risk profile (grade 2 arterial hypertension with ≥3 CV risk factors), preclinical organ damage.

Workup

For this patient the provisional diagnosis is of "resistant hypertension", since the patient is not at BP target (BP is largely ≥140/90 mmHg) despite the use of three drugs at full doses. True resistant hypertension at that time was not confirmed, since home BP values were particularly variable, probably due to incorrect measurement, and an ambulatory BP monitoring had never been performed.

During the visit the importance of lifestyle changes, of the reduction of alcohol consumption and of a healthier diet were stressed.

Treatment Evaluation

✓ Ongoing antihypertensive treatment was continued. A statin was added.

Treatment Prescribed

– Ramipril 10 mg once daily (h 08.00)
– Atenolol 100 mg once daily (h 08.00)
– Hydrochlorothiazide 25 mg (h 8.00)
– Atorvastatin 40 mg (h 20.00)

Prescriptions

✓ Lifestyle changes were recommended, with particular emphasis on a low-calorie, low-fat and low-salt diet, rich in fruit and vegetables.

✓ Adherence to treatment was recommended.

✓ Twenty-four-hour ambulatory blood pressure monitoring was scheduled within 2 weeks.

✓ The patient was instructed to measure BP at home with a standardized approach (sitting for at least 5 min in a quiet room, repeating measurements 2–3 times in each occasion and recording the mean value).

✓ An echocardiogram and measurement of albuminuria, serum TSH and urinary cortisol were also prescribed.

6.2   Follow-Up (Visit 1) at 4 Weeks

At follow-up visit, the patient was asymptomatic, with the exception of the known mild exercise intolerance.

He had started more frequent measurements of BP values. Mean values at home were still elevated.

His lifestyle did not seem to have been significantly improved, according to his wife (still high alcohol intake and low physical activity, unhealthy diets).

Body weight was unchanged.

The patient declared to be adherent to antihypertensive treatment.

No drug-related side effects were reported.

Physical Examination

- Weight: 110 kg
- Height: 175 cm
- Body mass index (BMI): 36 kg/m^2
- Waist circumference: 120 cm
- Resting pulse: regular rhythm with normal heart rate (82 beats/min)
- Other clinical parameters substantially unchanged

Blood Pressure Profile

- Home BP (average): 162/74 mmHg
- Office sitting BP: 172/82 mmHg
- Standing BP: 166/90 mmHg at 1 min

The ambulatory blood pressure monitoring profile showed increased 24 h BP, with values above the suggested thresholds both during the day and the night.

- 24-h BP: 169/70 mmHg
- Daytime BP: 169/69 mmHg
- Night-time BP: 170/72 mmHg

The analysis 24-h blood pressure profile shows an increased BP variability, as indicated by the standard deviation of BP values (standard deviation of 24 h night-time SBP: 14.6).

Day-to-night BP reduction was absent. Therefore, the ambulatory blood pressure monitoring showed features associated to increased CV risk [2].

Figure 6.3 shows the 24-h ambulatory blood pressure profile.

Polysomnography was performed, and sleep apnoea was excluded.

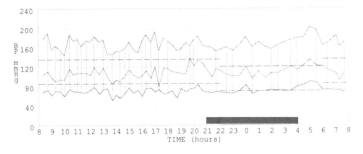

FIGURE 6.3 24-hour blood pressure profile at first follow-up visit

Current Treatment

- Ramipril 10 mg once daily (h 08.00)
- Atenolol 100 mg once daily (h 08.00)
- Hydrochlorothiazide 25 mg (h 8.00)
- Atorvastatin 40 mg (h 20.00)

Haematological Profile

- Glycosylated haemoglobin was 42 mmol/mol (6 %).
- Albuminuria: albumin/creatinine ratio: 24 mg/g.
- Serum TSH normal.
- 24 h urinary cortisol 15 μg/24 h.

Echocardiogram

The echocardiogram showed non-dilated eccentric left ventricular hypertrophy (LVMI 59 g/m$^{2.7}$, RWT 0.40) (Fig. 6.4), with preserved systolic function. Left atrial volume was normal (25 mL/BSA). There are no signs of increased LV filling pressures (TDI: E/E^1 6.0).

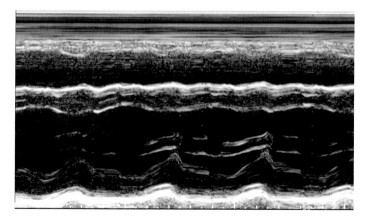

FIGURE 6.4 Echocardiogram

Diagnosis

Which is the correct diagnosis?
Possible answers are:

1. Isolated office hypertension
2. Sleep apnoea syndrome with arterial hypertension
3. Hypertension in Cushing syndrome
4. Hypertension, resistant to treatment due to the presence of comorbidities and inadequate adherence to lifestyle changes (excessive intake of alcohol, calories and salt)

Diagnosis: hypertension (grade 2, high CV risk) resistant to treatment (due to comorbidities—obesity—and to low adherence to healthy lifestyle).

Treatment Evaluation

✓ Treatment with a combination of four drugs was initiated. A potent, long-acting angiotensin receptor blocker (ARB) at full dose was initiated, together with a potent and long-acting calcium antagonist at medium dose (single-pill combination). A fixed, single-pill combination of a new-generation beta blocker and a diuretic was also added.

Treatment Prescribed

– Olmesartan 40 mg/amlodipine 5 mg OD at 8
– Nebivolol 5 mg/hydrochlorothiazide 25 mg OD at 8
– Atorvastatin 40 mg at 20

Prescriptions

✓ A new interview with the patient was done, in order to try to obtain adherence to lifestyle.

✓ The patient was sent to a dietician.

✓ Regular physical activity and low caloric intake were recommended.

✓ Periodical BP evaluation at home according to recommendations from current guidelines.

✓ Adherence to treatment was recommended (further discussion on the importance of adherence to the therapeutic plan in order to maximize cardiovascular protection).

6.3   Follow-Up (Visit 2) at 2 Months

At follow-up visit at 2 months, the patient was well and asymptomatic.

He had only partially modified his lifestyle, having reduced alcohol intake to about ¾ of litre of wine per day and had stopped taking hard drinks. He was still sedentary but he had slightly increased physical activity. His diet was substantially unchanged.

His weight was only slightly reduced (−3 kg from the first visit).

Self-reported adherence to treatment was good.

He described the reduction of the number of pills was a pleasant novelty.

No drug-related side effects were reported.

Physical Examination

- Height: 175 cm
- Weight: 107 kg
- Body mass index (BMI): 35 kg/m^2
- Waist circumference: 117 cm

- Resting pulse: regular rhythm with normal heart rate (80 beats/min)
- No ankle oedema
- Other clinical parameters substantially unchanged

Blood Pressure Profile

- Home BP (average): 144/74 mmHg
- Office sitting BP: 156/78 mmHg
- Standing BP: 154/82 mmHg at 1 min

Current Treatment

– Olmesartan 40 mg/amlodipine 5 mg OD at 8 am
– Nebivolol 5 mg/hydrochlorothiazide 25 mg OD at 8 am
– Atorvastatin 40 mg at 20

Treatment Evaluation

✓ The combination of an ARB, a calcium antagonist, a beta blocker and a diuretic was maintained.
✓ The dosage of the calcium antagonist was increased, since no side effect had been reported by the patient.

Treatment Prescribed

– Olmesartan 40 mg/amlodipine 10 mg OD at 8 am
– Nebivolol 5 mg/hydrochlorothiazide 25 mg OD at 8 am
– Atorvastatin 40 mg at 20

Prescriptions

✓ The medical staff reinforced the recommendations on lifestyle and tried to educate the patient about correct lifestyle.

✓ Home BP measurement was recommended, together with periodic BP measurement at the office of the general practitioner.
✓ A further visit after 40 days was scheduled.

6.4   Follow-Up (Visit 3) at 3 Months

The patient was seen at the Hypertension Clinic for a control visit.

He was asymptomatic, and his mild exercise intolerance was improved.

His lifestyle was discretely improved.

He was continuing moderate physical activity. His diet was still not optimal, but he had reduced alcohol intake. In fact, he was drinking about ½ litre of wine per day (no other alcoholic drinks in his diet).

Physical Examination

- Height: 175 cm
- Weight: 105 kg
- Body mass index (BMI): 34 kg/m^2
- Resting pulse: regular rhythm with normal heart rate (72 beats/min)
- Minimal ankle oedema
- Other clinical parameters substantially unchanged

Haematological Profile

- Electrolytes: potassium, 4.9 mEq/L
- Renal function: creatinine, 1.3 eGFR CKD-EPI 56 mL/min/1.73 m^2
- Fasting plasma glucose: 110 mg/dL
- Fasting lipids: total cholesterol 170 mg/dL, HDL 42 mg/dL, triglycerides 125 mg/dL, LDL 103 mg/dL

Blood Pressure Profile

- Home BP (average): 140/70 mmHg
- Office sitting BP: 148/76 mmHg
- Standing BP: 148/80 mmHg at 1 min

    The electrocardiogram was substantially unchanged.

Current Treatment

- Olmesartan 40 mg/amlodipine 10 mg OD at 8 am
- Nebivolol 5 mg/hydrochlorothiazide 25 mg OD at 8 am
- Atorvastatin 40 mg at 20

Treatment Evaluation

✓ The double-fixed, single-pill combination of ARB/calcium antagonist and beta blocker/diuretic was left unchanged, and doxazosin was added.

Treatment Prescribed

– Olmesartan 40 mg/amlodipine 10 mg OD at 8 am
– Nebivolol 5 mg/hydrochlorothiazide 25 mg OD at 8 am
– Doxazosin 2 mg OD in the evening (decrease dosage to 1 mg for the first 3 evenings)
– Atorvastatin 40 mg at 20

Prescriptions

✓ Lifestyle recommendations were reinforced (regular physical activity and low caloric intake, increase fruit and vegetables, reduce sodium intake).
✓ Further appointments with the dietician were arranged.
✓ BP measurements at home were recommended.

6.5 Follow-Up (Visit 4) at 6 Months

The patient was seen for the fourth time at the Hypertension Clinic in 6 months.

He was asymptomatic, and his mild exercise intolerance was improved.

His lifestyle was discretely improved.

He was continuing moderate physical activity. His diet was still not optimal, but he had reduced alcohol intake. In fact, he was drinking about ½ litre of wine per day (no other alcoholic drinks in his diet).

Physical Examination

- Height: 175 cm
- Weight: 100 kg
- Body mass index (BMI): 32.6 kg/m^2
- Resting pulse: regular rhythm with normal heart rate (72 beats/min)
- Mild ankle oedema

Blood Pressure Profile

- Home BP (average): 135/70 mmHg
- Office sitting BP: 144/74 mmHg
- Standing BP: 142/78 mmHg at 1 min

Current Treatment

- Olmesartan 40 mg/amlodipine 10 mg OD at 8 am
- Nebivolol 5 mg/hydrochlorothiazide 25 mg OD at 8 am
- Doxazosin 2 mg OD in the evening
- Atorvastatin 40 mg in the evening

Treatment Evaluation

✓ The fixed, single-pill combination of ACE inhibitor, calcium antagonist and diuretic was left unchanged, and doxazosin dosage was increased.

Treatment Prescribed

– Olmesartan 40 mg/amlodipine 10 mg OD at 8 am
– Nebivolol 5 mg/hydrochlorothiazide 25 mg OD at 8 am
– Doxazosin 4 mg OD in the evening
– Atorvastatin 40 mg in the evening

Prescriptions

✓ Lifestyle recommendations were reinforced (regular physical activity and low caloric intake, increase fruit and vegetables, reduce sodium intake).
✓ BP measurements at home were recommended.
✓ The patient was told to undergo an echocardiogram, an electrocardiogram and an ABPM within 6–12 months

6.6   Discussion

This clinical case describes a common condition: in everyday practice, hypertensive patients do not infrequently fail to obtain BP control due to the presence of comorbidities [1, 3]. In these patients, when BP is not controlled, the initial workup should include more accurate evaluation of BP values with the aim of identifying patients with "truly resistant" hypertension [1]. Interestingly, the finding of left ventricular hypertrophy in the patient described in this clinical case supports a sustained elevation of BP values. In addition, the mild reduction of eGFR, together with borderline values of urinary albumin excretion, indicates initial hypertensive renal damage. A number of studies [4, 5] have shown that patients with true resistant hypertension have a higher prevalence of electrocardiographic and echocardiographic left ventricular hypertrophy, as well as of vascular and renal damage, which may explain the increase in CV risk in these patients but may also render hypertension more difficult to control.

Indeed, other aspects might explain the difficulties in obtaining BP control in this patient. Firstly, despite the favourable effect exerted by moderate alcohol intake on the cardiovascular system, excessive alcohol intake (including binge drinking) is associated to elevation of BP values and treatment-resistant hypertension. Therefore, excessive alcohol intake should be carefully verified in all patients with resistant hypertension, and, when present, efforts should be made in order to stop alcohol intake [1]. Secondly, in this patient the presence of obesity seems to play a major role in treatment resistance. At the first visit, grade 2 obesity was diagnosed, and a significant increase in abdominal circumference was recorded. Obesity and overweight are common in patients with BP elevation, being present in about 75 % of the hypertensive patients seen by general practitioners or specialists [6]. Several abnormalities might explain the development or maintenance of arterial hypertension in obese and overweight subjects [7]. Overactivity of the sympathetic nervous system has been described in obesity, both in animal models and in humans. In addition, evidence has accumulated in support of an activation of the renin-angiotensin system in obesity. Furthermore, several alterations in renal structure and function can cause abnormal sodium retention and raise arterial pressure in obese and overweight patients. An important aspect is also represented by sleep apnoea [1, 7, 8], which is common in obese patients and which is strictly associated to hypertension (and in particular, but not only, to nocturnal hypertension) and resistance to treatment. Elevated BP values during the night should raise the suspicion of sleep apnoea syndrome, especially in obese patients. An accurate assessment of symptoms such as snoring and daytime sleepiness is mandatory in patients with resistant hypertension, possibly including the use of validated questionnaires.

Continuous positive airway pressure therapy is a useful tool for reducing obstructive sleep apnoea, and the available data seem to indicate that it is also capable of reducing BP values in these patients, in particular in those with daytime sleepiness; data on the possible reduction of cardiovascular events are, however, scarce.

In this patient sleep apnoea was ruled out by polysomnography. The therapeutic strategy chosen was based on a combination of full doses of a long-acting ARB, a calcium channel blocker, a diuretic, a vasodilating beta blocker and doxazosin, with the use of fixed-dose combinations, in order to maximize adherence to treatment. The choice of substituting ramipril with olmesartan was dictated by the observed increase in BP values in the last hours of the night-time period: in fact in elderly hypertensive patients, olmesartan is more effective in reducing 24-h BP values [9], and this effect has been found particularly evident in the last hours before drug intake. A mineralocorticoid receptor antagonist might have been theoretically a reasonable choice for this patient [1, 8], given the demonstrated efficacy of this class of drugs in resistant hypertension and the possible contribution of increased aldosterone levels in the elevation of BP values in obese patients. However, the option was discarded, due to the presence of potassium levels in the high-normal range, and doxazosin was therefore prescribed, another drug with demonstrated effectiveness in patients with resistant hypertension.

Indeed, the most effective strategy for reaching BP control in this patient would have been represented by a clear change in lifestyle, with complete cessation of alcohol intake, limitation of dietary salt, increased physical activity and weight control. However, it is well known that weight control is not easy to be obtained in everyday practice and that overweight and obesity significantly contribute to increase cardiovascular risk in hypertensive patients.

Take-Home Messages

- Overweight and obesity are common in hypertensive patients, being present in about 75 % of hypertensive patients visited by medical practitioners and internists.
- Obesity, often associated to excessive salt and/or alcohol intake, is not infrequent as a cause of secondary resistant hypertension.
- In hypertensive patients, ethanol consumption should not exceed 20–30 g in males and 10–20 g in women per day.
- When resistant hypertension and obesity coexist, the most effective strategy for reaching BP control is represented by changes in lifestyle, with limitation (possibly cessation) of alcohol intake, limitation of dietary salt and increased physical activity.
- When not contraindicated, mineralocorticoid receptor antagonists may be considered as third-line drugs in these patients, due to the possible role of increased aldosterone levels in the pathogenesis of resistance to treatment.

References

1. Mancia G, Fagard R, Narkiewicz K, Redon J, Zanchetti A, Bohm M, et al. 2013 ESH/ESC Guidelines for the management of arterial hypertension: the Task Force for the management of arterial hypertension of the European Society of Hypertension (ESH) and of the European Society of Cardiology (ESC). J Hypertens. 2013;31(7):1281–357.
2. Reboldi G, Angeli F, Verdecchia P. Ambulatory blood interpretation of pressure profile for risk stratification. Keep it simple. Hypertension. 2014;63:913–4.
3. Calhoun D, Booth J, Oparil S, Irvin M, Shimbo D, Lackland D, Howard G, Safford M, Muntner P. Refractory hypertension determination of prevalence, risk factors, and comorbidities in a large, population-based cohort. Hypertension. 2014;63:451–8.

4. De la Sierra A, Segura J, Banegas JR, et al. Clinical features of 8295 patients with resistant hypertension classified on the basis of ambulatory blood pressure monitoring. Hypertension. 2011;57: 898–902.
5. Muiesan ML, Salvetti M, Rizzoni D, Paini A, Agabiti-Rosei C, Aggiusti C, Agabiti RE. Resistant hypertension and target organ damage. Hypertens Res. 2013;36(6):485–91.
6. Bramlage P, Pittrow D, Wittchen HU, Kirch W, Boehler S, Lehnert H, et al. Hypertension in overweight and obese primary care patients is highly prevalent and poorly controlled. Am J Hypertens. 2004;17:904–10.
7. Rojas E, Velasco M, Bermúdez V, Israili Z, Bolli P. Targeting hypertension in patients with cardiorenal metabolic syndrome. Curr Hypertens Rep. 2012;14(5):397–402.
8. Jordan J, Schlaich M, Redon J, Narkiewicz K, Luft FC, Grassi G, Dixon J, Lambert G, Engeli S, for the European Society of Hypertension Working Group on Obesity and the Australian and New Zealand Obesity Society. European society of hypertension working group on obesity: obesity drugs and cardiovascular outcomes. J Hypertens. 2011;29:189–93.
9. Malacco E, Omboni S, Volpe M, Auteri A, Zanchetti A, ESPORT Study Group. Antihypertensive efficacy and safety of olmesartan medoxomil and ramipril in elderly patients with mild to moderate essential hypertension: the ESPORT study. J Hypertens. 2010;28(11):2342–50.

Printed in the United States
By Bookmasters